Reading Literature and Chronic Pain

Reading Literature and Chronic Pain

JOSIE BILLINGTON

BLOOMSBURY ACADEMIC
LONDON • NEW YORK • OXFORD • NEW DELHI • SYDNEY

BLOOMSBURY ACADEMIC
Bloomsbury Publishing Plc
50 Bedford Square, London, WC1B 3DP, UK
1385 Broadway, New York, NY 10018, USA
29 Earlsfort Terrace, Dublin 2, Ireland

BLOOMSBURY, BLOOMSBURY ACADEMIC and the Diana logo are trademarks of Bloomsbury Publishing Plc

First published in Great Britain 2025

Cover design: Eleanor Rose
Cover image © Vince Cavataio/Getty Images

A catalogue record for this book is available from the British Library.

Library of Congress Cataloging-in-Publication Data

Names: Billington, Josie, 1961- author.
Title: Reading literature and chronic pain / Josie Billington.
Description: London ; New York : Bloomsbury Academic, 2025. | Includes bibliographical references and index. | Summary: "This valuable and insightful study into chronic pain and its treatment advances a striking analysis of the complex phenomenon of chronic pain, also attesting to the importance of the medical humanities in addressing urgent questions that medical science alone cannot resolve. Based on unique empirical research with people who are living with chronic pain, this book is the first of its kind to demonstrate the value of literature and literary reading both as a discourse for understanding pain and as an intervention in its treatment"– Provided by publisher.
Identifiers: LCCN 2024050795 (print) | LCCN 2024050796 (ebook) | ISBN 9781350270251 (paperback) | ISBN 9781350270213 (hardback) | ISBN 9781350270237 (epub) | ISBN 9781350270220 (ebook)
Subjects: LCSH: Chronic pain–Treatment. | Bibliotherapy. | Group reading–Therapeutic use.
Classification: LCC RB127.5.C48 B55 2025 (print) | LCC RB127.5.C48 (ebook) | DDC 616/.0472–dc23/eng/20250212
LC record available at https://lccn.loc.gov/2024050795
LC ebook record available at https://lccn.loc.gov/2024050796

ISBN: HB: 978-1- 3502-7021-3
PB: 978-1- 3502-7025-1
ePDF: 978-1- 3502-7022-0
eBook: 978-1- 3502-702-3

Typeset by Deanta Global Publishing Services, Chennai, India
Printed and bound in Great Britain

For product safety related questions contact productsafety@bloomsbury.com.

To find out more about our authors and books visit www.bloomsbury.com and sign up for our newsletters.

*Dedicated to all those who have contributed to the reading and pain
work documented here
and
in memory of James Ledson.*

Contents

PART III   Reading not talking: Pain, trauma, treatment

Preface

This book began life over a decade ago when I attended a Personalized Medicine conference at the University of Liverpool. Together with my colleagues in Medicine and Social Sciences, I (an English Literature specialist) had been invited to speak about a multidisciplinary study we had recently undertaken on the value of literary reading groups, as delivered by the UK charity The Reader, for people living with depression. We had demonstrated with scientific robustness that the combination of reading literary works, fiction and poetry, and the group experience had alleviated symptoms of depression to a 'statistically significant' degree. Participants had also reported that they found the reading group soothing and absorbing and were often surprised and grateful to rediscover powers of concentration and connectedness they felt they had lost.

Attending the conference were consultants from the pain clinic at the university hospital who subsequently invited the team to set up, via The Reader, a weekly reading group in the pain clinic and conduct an equivalent study. The rationale for this study was the fact that people with chronic pain have three times the average risk of developing psychiatric symptoms – usually mood or anxiety disorders – and depressed patients have three times the average risk of developing chronic pain. I knew nothing of the intimate connection between the two debilitating conditions. Frankly, I knew nothing (clinically speaking) about chronic pain. Neither had the opioid scandal in the United States yet broken to alert me (as it did many people) to the scale of this health problem. Given my background as a literature academic, this ignorance was unsurprising. What became alarming in the course of the study was how widespread this lack of knowledge was among newcomers to the medical profession. A third-year trainee medical student to whom I was teaching a session on this study as part of a Medical Humanities module exclaimed, 'Why don't I know anything about this?' The reason is simple, the pain consultants explained. 'Do you know how much is taught about chronic pain in medical schools? Nothing at all!' This is despite the fact that the condition is now widely acknowledged to affect as much as half the population in the western hemisphere.

The results from our study (as Part II will attest) were overwhelmingly positive in both statistical and qualitative terms. The evidence as to the value of literary reading for chronic pain was so convincing that it secured (to this day) continuous funding for the reading group and led to a change in practice at the clinic, where attending a literary reading group is now part of the pain management package alongside standard therapeutic interventions. I am still staggered by these consequences, even as I write about them, and despite the fact that I led and carried out much of the research. The question I hear the reader asking – 'How can something as apparently soft as reading fiction and poetry influence a condition as intractable as chronic pain?' – is in many ways still my own. The standard journal articles in which the findings were published necessarily concentrated on the phenomenon *that* reading helped pain sufferers, but left insufficient room and opportunity to ponder the bigger questions of *how* and *why* it did and does so, and what this says more widely about literary reading and about pain. This book is an attempt to correct that omission. As such, it involves quite a hefty 'backfill' project in the sense of finding out many of the things I did not know about chronic pain when my research unexpectedly intersected with this condition and, in particular, establishing which characteristics of chronic pain made it particularly susceptible to the power of literary reading. Exploration and discovery, therefore – the need to know and understand rather than comprehensive explanation – motivate large portions of this book. Thus, much of what follows in Part I will be common knowledge to health practitioners involved in treating pain, and at the same time appear incomplete as an account of the condition. My criterion for coverage has rested on my intuition about which aspects of the multi-dimensional experience of chronic pain literature has been 'treating', as it were. Above all, I do not, any more than fiction and poetry themselves purport to do, offer literary reading as some kind of miracle cure. Whatever it does, as demonstrated in the still partial evidence I am able to offer in this book, is more complicated than, and perhaps as needful as, a simple remedy.

One further preliminary. Chronic pain comprises or overlaps with a range of conditions, including fibromyalgia, back pain, migraine, irritable bowel syndrome and many others. In the course of the study we undertook, I had no access to participants' medical records and no knowledge of any more specific diagnosis than chronic pain. Consequently, in what follows, I do not distinguish 'types' of chronic pain. I do, nonetheless, draw on research evidence that relates to more particular diagnoses, especially in Chapter 1, where I judge the findings to have potential application to chronic pain in general. It is important to note, moreover, what much of the research cited reiterates: that chronic pain is not merely an accompanying symptom of another diagnosed condition but a condition in and of itself, with its own definition and taxonomy.

In Part I, I try to establish a broad picture of the medical and philosophical landscape which the literary reading experiment (unwittingly) entered. Influential twenty-first century studies of pain have come from a range of clinical, humanities and social science disciplines. These converge in calling for an understanding of pain that is multi-dimensional, in opposition and resistance to reductive biomedical models and treatments of pain. Yet the resonance and synergy across anthropological, clinical, cultural, historical and psychoanalytical perspectives, for example, are often hidden or unrecognized. In bringing these distinct discourses together, my intention is not to attempt a definitive synthesis. Rather, my aim is to bring these disciplines into live 'play' in order that I can draw on them freely in Part II, where I turn to the empirical study described above. This is because my experience of carrying out that empirical work has confirmed to me that all such perspectives, at various times and to differing extents, are relevant, even sometimes crucial.

Part II is the core of this book. It offers compelling vignettes or 'snapshots', in addition to extended case studies, of people living with chronic pain who read literature together, weekly, in a pain clinic at a UK hospital. These are based on video-recordings of reading group sessions over a period of six months gathered as part of a British Academy-funded study of literary reading and chronic pain. (The study was approved by a local NHS ethics committee. All participants gave informed consent. Pseudonyms are used throughout.) This part of the book demonstrates important intersections between the real-world research on literary reading and health which has taken place in the UK and the laboratory-based empirical studies in psychology, carried out concurrently in Europe and North America, on the psychological impact of literary reading. Indeed, this is a timely moment, two decades into the century which has seen the field of reading and health burgeon within a range of disciplines, to position these bodies of work in (albeit complex) relation to one another. Part II also uses key insights and concepts from psychology, social science and psychoanalysis encountered in Part I as a lens through which to observe and understand reading processes and crucial reading moments. While individual readers are the focus of much of Part II, the final chapter draws on classic work in interpersonal and developmental psychology to explore the experience of shared group reading as a special mode of literary encounter.

Part III considers the implications of the theoretical survey in Part I and the empirical evidence in Part II for future understanding and treatment of chronic pain. It positions literary reading groups in close alignment with standard therapeutic approaches and psychosocial interventions for chronic pain, which target psychological 'stuckness'. In doing so, Part III enters into dialogue with contemporary psychiatric and neuroscientific work, which offers – with no axe to grind about the value of reading per se – some of the strongest grounds for, as well as challenges to, the idea of literature as cure.

This work owes an incalculable debt to colleagues, readers and study participants with whom I have worked, both on this and related projects, during the ten years of its development. My sincere and continuing thanks to my close and long-time valued colleagues at the University of Liverpool, Rhiannon Corcoran, Philip Davis, Chris Dowrick; and to colleagues, here and further afield, with whom I have worked more recently: Christopher Brown, Anne-Louise Humphreys, Jamie Lingwood, Don McCown, Neil Vickers. I owe huge thanks to my collaborators at The Reader charity and in the health service, for their invaluable moral, intellectual and material support, particularly Grace Farrington, Andrew Jones, Kate McDonnell, and also Amanda Boston, Clare Ellis, Jane Davis, Nicky Duirs, Kathryn Harney, Helen Wilson. Thanks are also due to the British Academy for funding the original study. I also wish to acknowledge my loving and ever supportive family, Tom, Matty, Sam and particularly on this occasion, Marianne (whose scholarly eye for detail has been a godsend). Finally, my strongest and warmest thanks go to the people who are the subject of this book and whose lives and pains, hearts and minds, it has been a unique privilege to think and feel alongside.

Chronic pain: Where is it? What is it?

Pain as symptom, experience and idea (past and present)

1

Chronic pain: The clinical picture

In the introduction to *Empire of Pain*, his magisterial and devastating account of the 'secret history of the Sackler dynasty', Patrick Radden Keefe describes how in 1996, drug manufacturer Purdue Pharma, a key source of the Sackler family fortune, marketed 'a groundbreaking drug, a powerful opioid painkiller called OxyContin, which was heralded as a revolutionary way to treat chronic pain'. A quarter of a century later, opioid-related overdoses had become 'the leading cause of accidental death in America', reaching 450,000 and 'accounting for more deaths than car accidents [and] gunshot wounds'. 'More Americans had lost their lives from opioid overdoses than had died in all the wars the country had fought since World War II.'[1] Data released in 2021 by the Centre for Disease Control and Prevention announced that 'Drug Overdose Deaths in the U.S. Top 100,000 Annually'.[2] A 2022 *Lancet* report predicted an additional 1.2 million deaths in North America by the end of this decade.[3]

To the scandalous marketing frauds, medical malpractices and breathtaking abuses of scientific integrity, which, as uncovered by Keefe, contributed to the formidable scale and depth of this tragedy, can be added the apparent total or wilful disregard for the state of knowledge in respect of chronic pain. Arthur Kleinman, Harvard professor of Global Health and Medicine, and director of the World Health Organisation report on mental health in the year before OxyContin was introduced, had written almost a decade earlier in his seminal work *The Illness Narratives*:

Understanding the meanings of pain and tracing out the dynamics of somatization in the fullness of the life of pain patients will show . . . that there is no such thing as *the* pain patient. . . . A single ideal treatment for all but a few atypical cases can also be readily shown to be a dangerous myth.[4]

Kleinman's deduction was based on twenty years' experience as an MD and the medical consensus that had emerged around pain in the United States and the UK in the second half of the twentieth century. Until the 1960s, chronic pain was understood to be essentially physiological in origin and in need, therefore, of physical treatments, chiefly medication and surgery. Among the influential developments in Western medicine and science which helped dislodge this view of chronic pain as being primarily a medical issue were two re-conceptualizations, one of health and one of pain. Firstly, George Engel's 'biopsychosocial model' of health proposed in 1977[5] 'was constructed to take into account the missing dimensions of the biomedical model'. It was offered as both a philosophy of and practical guide to clinical care, emphasizing a holistic approach which encompasses molecular, psychological and societal forces of influence; and above all recognizes the patient's subjective experience and sense of the meaning of illness as influencing the latter's presentation and course. 'Nothing exists in isolation. Whether a cell or a person, every system is influenced by the configuration of the systems of which each is a part.'[6] Secondly, Melzack's gate-control theory of pain, advanced in the 1960s, replaced the dominant theory of pain as transmitted outside-in, from peripheral somatic stimulation to the nervous system and brain, by proposing that the experience of pain is modulated by nerve impulses that descend from the brain and inhibit or facilitate painful sensation. This was the foundation for what is now known as the 'neuromatrix' theory of pain,[7] which concludes that pain (as with all perceptual experiences) is the result of brain activation across a widely distributed neural network, produced by a convergence of cognitive, emotional and sensory inputs and may occur in the absence of the latter. Accordingly, a biopsychosocial understanding has come to predominate among professionals and scientists of the western hemisphere who regard chronic pain as 'a multidimensional, dynamic interaction among physiological, psychological, and social factors that reciprocally influence each other'.[8] As we shall see, results emerging from the surge in neuroimaging in recent decades have served to confirm that chronic pain is complex in origin and highly influenced, as an experience, by individual pathophysiology, psychological state, emotional factors and social milieu. The biological evidence itself points to non-biological influences on pain and the need for approaches that are holistic, not narrowly pharmacological, in symptom management.

This orientation is reflected in the most widely accepted, official definition of chronic pain in use today, provided by the International Association for the Study of Pain: 'An unpleasant sensory and emotional experience associated with, or resembling that associated with, actual or potential tissue damage'[9] which persists or recurs for longer than three months. 'Sensory *and emotional*'; 'actual *or potential*'. These adjectives are key, as the pain consultants I worked with explained: *Defining pain as an 'emotional' experience is crucial.*

Arguably, if you do not have an emotional response to your pain, then you are probably not suffering from pain. It is not a merely physical sensation like hot or cold or a vibration. If you take the emotion out of pain, it's not pain anymore. Furthermore, it is often not simply the case that *something is damaged, it hurts, you rest or treat it, it gets better. For some reason, in certain people's nervous systems, the pain stays; it does not get better with tissue healing. The pain may or may not have been triggered by tissue damage in the first place. Either way, chronic pain sufferers are experiencing something that is totally 'inappropriate' – they're getting pain which is not justified by and not related to any tissue damage.* What the adjectives used in the standard definition ('emotional', 'potential') gesture towards is the one certainty about chronic pain: that it is a subjective phenomenon: *Only the sufferer can 'measure' the pain – by explaining where the pain is, how intense it is, how long it lasts, its quality, impact, meaning. Measuring pain on a scale of 1–10 is virtually meaningless to the chronic pain patient, for whom the pain fluctuates on a daily, weekly and monthly basis.*[10] A definition sufficiently loose to allow for multiple influences and experiences of chronic pain does not guarantee satisfactory outcomes at the level of care, however. Officially defined by the duration of its symptoms, chronic pain is 'in reality, a state of physical suffering strongly associated with feelings of anxiety, depression and despair'.[11] It is one of the most common symptoms reported in Western healthcare,[12] and one of the most resistant to successful treatment. Drugs cannot efficiently target a condition where the relation of pain to biology is variable and unreliable (though this has not prevented the widespread use of highly addictive opioids). It is widely acknowledged that alternatives to conventional treatments are necessary to take into account psychosocial and psycho-emotional dimensions of pain, and the current research base supports the use of psychological therapies. But there remains a 'desperate need'[13] for effective therapies to be embedded in healthcare.

Let me sketch the disturbing potential scenario in the UK if that need is not met. The paradigm or (fore-)'shadow' story is the current national situation regarding the treatment of depression, which, as mentioned already and as detailed shortly, is closely allied, and usually co-morbid, with chronic pain. In the ten years preceding the publication of the study on which this book is based, the number of antidepressants prescribed in the UK had more than doubled (from 33.7 to 64.7 million).[14] This was part of a global trend consequent upon the increasing configuration of a wide spectrum of emotional experiences as constituting mental health issues in need of medical treatment. The emphasis on characterizing common human sorrows as illness, or on 'medicalising unhappiness'[15] – authorized in particular by the powerfully influential dictionary of symptoms published by American Psychiatry, the *Diagnostic and Statistical Manual of Mental Disorders* (*DSM*) (whose role in relation to chronic pain I detail in Chapter 4) – was the originating impulse for the reading and depression study I refer to in the Preface.[16] But this decidedly cultural tendency cannot alone account for the large regional variation across the UK, which saw the prescribing of antidepressant medication over-represented in areas of socio-economic deprivation in the North and East of England. The highest prescribing district in the country was located in North West England (the region in which the study to which I devote Part II took place).[17] It is well documented that the prevalence of reported mental health problems in England in this decade was closely associated with the economic recession consequent upon the global financial crisis of 2008 and the welfare policy reforms which it engendered.[18] (The association of depression and deprivation remains highest, incidentally, in North West England in recent studies.[19]) Felicity Thomas's near-contemporaneous work on mental health and austerity draws urgent attention to the manifold implications of the disproportionately high levels of prescribing and use of psychiatric drugs within low-income communities, chief among which is 'the pathologisation and medicalisation of poverty and disadvantage'. While 'distress is an unexceptional and expected reaction to difficult circumstances, the chances of this distress being diagnosed and treated as mental illness are now extremely high'. On the one hand, there is increasing pressure on GPs to provide for social care as well as medical needs, as wider statutory services are cut to the bone; and to do so within their own restrictions on time, financial resources and (hence) treatment options, in a context where prescribing medication may already be embedded in their primary care practice. On the other hand, 'in situations where people's social standing and access to welfare support are increasingly and intrinsically connected to their health status and their ability to evidence sickness . . . dominant biomedical narratives inherent within current mental health and welfare strategies may themselves be shaping experiences of, and responses to, mental health and wellbeing amongst low-income groups in the UK'.[20] When the GP is the only place to turn for welfare support – emotionally and socially – the orientation of distress towards medical diagnosis and treatment is likely to be the patient's as much as the doctor's. All the while, the chances of distress being thereby intensified, rather than alleviated, multiply. Established accounts of the association of poverty and mental ill health identify this reciprocity: hunger, debt and poor housing drive both mental health issues and the search for medical help, and people with a diagnosis of mental illness are disproportionately represented among the insecurely employed and homeless populations. Above all, the efficacy of the antidepressant treatment they receive is highly dubious: while the effect on mild depression is negligible and carries the risk of side effects such as suicidal ideation, long-term use (approximately half of the people on antidepressants are users of two years' standing or more) can aggravate relatively minor episodes of mental ill health, establish vulnerability to future depressive episodes and trigger new symptoms (of psychosis, for example). In a climate which discourages reassessment of treatment decisions, or support with withdrawal-related issues, an epidemic of dependency happens almost by default. 'Seeking greater understanding of the possibilities of establishing practice that takes a more holistic approach to understanding the complex interplay between coexisting physical, mental and social problems[21] is therefore vital if the realities of people's lives are to be more effectively supported in the coming years.'[22] Thomas's recommendation echoes precisely the view of the pain consultants in this study, who often felt they should not use the word 'pain' for these patients. *What they have is suffering. They do not have a localized symptoms. Their whole lives are globally awful.*

In the remainder of this chapter, I endeavour to give an insight, albeit of a generalized rather than individualized kind, into the nature of this suffering. I do so to underscore the complexity of the condition and the challenge it offers to the claim of this book: that literary reading can be a valuable source of life support for people living with chronic pain. The intention is also to provide an outline of the biopsychosocial understanding of chronic pain which formed the clinical context for the reading study which I treat in detail in Part II. Not everything, it is true, will apply directly to the people who took part in the study which is at the centre of Part II and this book. But as I have, and can give, no specific details of the participants' clinical backgrounds, and no more of their personal biographies than they chose to reveal, this composite picture is intended to supply as rich a picture of chronic pain, considered as a clinical condition, as I am able to give.

A note on terms and foci. I use the term 'clinical' here for two reasons: firstly, because the reading experiment, as will become clear, was conducted entirely within a clinical context, a weekly pain clinic at a UK NHS hospital; secondly, and relatedly, because the adjective clearly identifies the sociocultural specificity of this account of chronic pain – as primarily determined, that is to say, by Western (principally US and UK-focused) medical understandings and practices. My recounting of this model of pain does not amount to uncritical acceptance of it. As I have indicated already, the pain clinicians with whom I worked were by no means (quite the contrary) wedded to a reductively biomedical understanding of chronic pain; and, as we shall see shortly, the authorized clinical understanding of chronic pain in which they operated integrates psychological and sociological perspectives within its overarching clinical frame. But for both patients and doctors (as Thomas's account of UK experiences of treated depression helps to underscore), this clinical framework is a crucial and central reference point. So will it be for the health workers, and the pain sufferers, who, I hope, will compose part of the readership for this book. I recount this model in detail above all in recognition that the alternative to biomedical intervention which this book proposes – alternatives, I reiterate, which are 'desperately' and urgently needed – must, at the present time at least, gain traction and acceptance within those very practices. I return to this issue at the close of this chapter and at the end of the book.

There are, moreover, epistemological reasons for my emphasis on UK and US models and practices, given the strong historical and theoretical grounds for regarding the chronicity of chronic illness as a *construct* as well as a *symptom* of Western modernity. 'The classificatory term "chronic" [deriving from the Greek term for time, *chronos*]' emerged in the United States during the postwar period of the 1950s, when 'new appointment systems in general practice and effective patient records were established'. In the interests of rendering health care practice 'efficient . . . economical and effective', there was 'a postwar invasion of assessors, who counted and calculated time [according to] the same logic of capitalist production'. 'Thus, "chronicity", as it was conceived in the 1950s, was far from an ahistorical and essential phenomenon but, instead, related to specific sociohistorical discourses and practices' and their 'temporal logic'.[23] The relation of chronic illness to medical temporalities, and to lived experience of time, is an issue to which I will return frequently in Part II.

There is, furthermore, a large body of thinking and (social) theory which configures 'the chronic' as a particular way of experiencing the contemporary moment in the UK and the United States. The rise in rates of chronic illness, alongside the decline in the prevalence of epidemic infectious diseases (polio, tetanus), 'becomes a symbol of arrival for many industrializing nations'. 'Modern life imprints on the body.'[24] Some imprints have a long history, including the accelerated production of food and slow environmental changes to climate and plant and animal life. Some are felt directly by and in the body, like 'the permanent drain on our energy reserves' attendant, at one extreme, on the ubiquity and constancy of information and communication technologies and, at another, on 'the imperative to be productive' when being so has been 'stripped entirely of [any] spiritual dimension'.[25] Other harms are imprinted by the 'cultural baggage that attends the capitalist world economy',[26] the demands, for example, which individualism places upon the (apparently) autonomous self. In his Foucauldian account of depression, French sociologist Alain Ehrenberg traces a trend from the 1960s (when the institutional functions of socialization exercised by the family were, to a great extent, carried over to the school) when 'self-control, flexibility of mind and feeling and the capacity for action' were the new 'rules' of social conformity. The consequence was that 'each individual had to be up to the task of constantly adapting to a changing world that was losing its stable shape . . . to take on the job of choosing and deciding everything'. Depression is 'the pathology of a society whose norm . . . is based on responsibility and initiative' and wherein 'the individual is confronted with a pathology of inadequacy'.[27] A diagnosis of depression, as we have seen, 'privatises and psychologises' the 'suffering society creates'.[28] Chronic physical conditions (as we shall also see) are often framed somewhat differently 'within a moral narrative of lifestyle excess'[29] in respect, for example, of diet, alcohol consumption, smoking and inactivity. It is a discourse which, insofar as it is driven by the commercial interests of the drugs companies and private medicine, 'keeps intervention efforts focused on diagnosis' and 'long-term expensive fixes', rather than on 'the structures of a healthy society that undergird population health'. The chronic 'pathology' of Western capitalist economy is thus 'invisibly tied to biomedical meaning systems'.[30] A counter-discourse among global health scholars, in resistance to the exploitative internationalization of the Western healthcare market and rhetoric, has begun to ask what high-income countries can valuably learn from indigenous experiences and care practices in respect of chronic illness in low-income countries.[31] Such important and rewarding exploration goes beyond the scope of the current study. But the clinical narrative offered below is not ignorant of, even as it inevitably in part reproduces, the shaping influences of Western biomedical hegemony.

The psychology of pain

Chronic pain and depression

As indicated already, the development of a long-term pain condition is associated with a significant ('severalfold'[32]) increased risk of developing distress and anxiety symptoms and pain is a powerful predictor of depression relative to key demographic variables.[33] Depression rates, moreover, seem to be higher in chronic pain than in other chronic medical populations.[34] Even taking into account the wide variability in means of assessing depression, it appears that having a chronic condition does not itself sufficiently account for the development of depression. Rather, there are aspects particular to chronic *pain* which make depression a lamentably common and, as will become abundantly apparent, wholly unsurprising sequela.

As we have seen, nonetheless, 'current diagnostic and treatment frameworks assume a separation of problems that are seen to require quite distinct treatment pathways' which 'in practice . . . has direct implications not only for individual health and wellbeing outcomes, but for broader debates around the structure and economics of healthcare provision'.[35] This in turn has led to the 'silent epidemic' of chronic pain, and its 'embeddedness in society', becoming a 'blind spot' in a socio-theoretical 'diagnosis of a depressed society' and has occluded the degree to which depression and chronic pain are 'two sides of the same coin':

> If one does not want to regard it as a mere coincidence that both diseases share similarities phenomenally and in their respective prevalence [then] one needs to expand the *Zeitdiagnose* [socio-critical narrative] of a depressed society by integrating chronic pain into it. . . . [It must be recognized] that *the depressed society also suffers from chronic pain.*[36]

What follows explicates the degree to which the clinical evidence itself, even as it proceeds from, and often leads to, a more medical orientation and narrative, gives strong grounds for the separation of chronic pain and depression as untenable.

The most recent *Diagnostic and Statistical Manual of Mental Disorders* (DSM-5)[37] defines Major Depressive Disorder (or Clinical Depression) according to the experience of at least five of the following symptoms (including the first or second) over a two-week period: depressed mood, loss of interest/pleasure, weight loss or gain, insomnia or hypersomnia, psychomotor agitation or retardation (excessive or slowed thought or physical movement), fatigue or loss of energy, feeling worthless or excessive/inappropriate guilt, decreased concentration/decisiveness, recurrent thoughts of death/suicide. Bearing in mind that the official definition of chronic pain is its persistence for at least three months, and that insomnia,[38] immobility[39] and weight change[40] are de facto accompaniments of many types of chronic pain with well-documented knock-on effects on functioning, concentration, mood and overall quality of life,[41] it is difficult to imagine how the avoidance of many of these symptoms, together over a sustained period, would even be possible.

Standard cognitive behavioural models of depression also appear to apply with particular relevance to chronic pain. One account of depression posits 'attributional style' – how the 'perceiver uses information to arrive at causal explanations for events'[42] – as a key vulnerability factor. The theory of attributional style originated from Martin Seligman's model of 'learned helplessness' in which, in response to recurrent exposure to painful stimuli against which he or she is powerless, an individual develops the expectation of not being able to direct future outcomes through personal actions. Helplessness, that is to say, 'does not result from trauma per se'.[43] It is a form of negative learning from experience, in which the waning of motivation to respond in the face of aversive events, and the inability to recognize where response has worked, results in the emotional affective disturbance of depression. In the fully developed model, what mediates between the perceived loss of control and depression is the cause to which the helplessness is attributed. Here is one outline of the trajectory from chronic pain to depression, using this model.

> [When] chronic pain sufferers ask themselves why they have pain or why they are not able to control their pain . . . [they may have a pre-existing propensity to] make attributions that are: *internal* (e.g. 'It's my fault that I hurt myself and now have this back problem', or 'I can't tolerate the pain because I'm a weak person'); *stable* (e.g. 'I've always been prone to accidents', or 'Every time I try to exercise, my back ends up feeling worse'); and *global* (e.g. 'This is one more thing to add to my problems', 'No matter what I do, my back is killing me', or 'I can't control my pain because nothing in my life seems controllable'). These helplessness beliefs could conceivably generalize to other domains of living. In time, the helplessness may lead to a dysphoric mood, decreased motivation to cope with pain, and other deficits associated with Major Depressive Disorder.[44] (My emphases)

Such propensities are likely to be exercised all the more in the case of an adverse and painful event for which external explanations do not readily exist, which is by definition not transient or intermittent but abiding or 'stable', and which results in consequences that affect a whole life (including job loss, impact on family relationships and friendships and inability to pursue hobbies and interests[45]). Where pre-existing propensities do exist, chronic pain is a particularly powerful trigger for depression. In Aaron T. Beck's widely influential cognitive model of depression, the 'systematic cognitive bias', whereby people in the grip of depression attend to 'negative aspects of experience . . . blocking positive events and memories', is produced by 'highly charged dysfunctional attitudes or beliefs' in relation to self that 'hijack' the information processing system and produce selectivity of attention, recall, and interpretation and cognitive distortion.[46] Beck's model proposes that these dysfunctional attitudes are embedded within cognitive structures, or schemas, formed in response to adverse developmental experiences. When activated by stressful life events, the schemas produce a negative attentional bias and distorted global perception of reality, as well as depressive symptoms (withdrawal, inactivity, loss of motivation), which symptoms are themselves subjected to negative evaluation ('I am lazy/worthless/useless'). 'Thus, the depressive constellation consists of a continuous feedback loop with negative interpretations and attentional biases, subjective and behavioural symptoms, reinforcing each other.'[47] Chronic pain, it has been suggested, is a unique stressor in this regard, which may 'more specifically match or more intensely and recurrently activate cognitive vulnerabilities for depression' than other chronic symptoms. That is to say, pain activates negative schema and a correspondingly negative response to the pain itself, thereby increasing pain's magnitude and reactivating negative cognition, such that pain and depressive symptoms are 'dynamic, reciprocal, self-perpetuating and escalating'.[48] In Beck's model, after repeated activation, the negative schemas are organized or 'locked' into a depressive mode, becoming relatively autonomous, and no longer as reactive to external stimuli and positive events in ways that might reduce negative thinking or mood.

> Attentional resources are disproportionately allocated from the external environment to internal experiences such as negative cognitions and sadness [and] resources are withdrawn from adaptive schemas such as coping and problem solving. . . . The negatively biased cognitive schemas function as (efficient but maladaptive) *automatic* information processors – rapid, involuntary, and sparing of resources.[49]

This quotation is from a paper in which Beck is specifically concerned with the ways in which his model of depression, first formulated in 1967,[50] might be reconfigured in light of this century's advances in neuroscience. The description bears a striking resemblance to the picture emerging from neurobiology of maladaptive automatic circuits which develop in chronic pain sufferers, whereby neuronal pathways between brain areas associated with negative affective cognition and pain perception become hardwired.[51] Consider that, in addition to these structural and procedural affinities between depression and chronic pain, the latter is inevitably often a catalyst for common stressors in relation to the former (marital breakdown, termination of employment, isolating immobility and confinement to the home), and that (as we shall see) responses from the medical profession often serve to invalidate sufferers' experience, and the potential for external factors to reinforce the internal negative feedback loop is all too apparent.

Of course, this does not only tell the story of why chronic pain is a strong risk factor for depression, but also of how depression is a strong risk factor for chronic pain.

While psychological symptomatology is often interpreted as a *consequence* of chronic pain, the active relationship between depression and pain means that psychological dysfunction is also a likely *determiner* of the development of chronic pain conditions.[52] Chronic pain both causes and results from poor mental health.[53] On the one hand, in the face of chronic pain, a psychological predisposition towards depression evolves into full-blown clinical depression. On the other hand, when depression precedes chronic pain, there is an increase in pain sensitivity and a lowering of pain tolerance thresholds, such that the likelihood of pain becoming chronic is strong. Importantly, depression, anxiety and distress are among the most potent and robust predictors of the *transition* from acute to chronic pain.

Before I consider some of the precise mechanisms of this transition in the next section, it is noteworthy that the synergy between pain and depression has important implications for treatment choices, or, more specifically, for what is (or ought to be) treated. Several studies have demonstrated that the use of antidepressants by patients with chronic pain and mood disorders produces fairly rapid analgesic benefits, which correlate exactly with relief of psychological distress.[54] Conversely, research evidence suggests that distress is associated with reduced benefit from a variety of pain treatments[55] contributing to up to a 50 per cent reduction in pain relief from oral opioids.[56] In view of the compelling evidence that patients with higher levels of anxiety and depression experience not only less benefit from surgical intervention but suffer more complications, increased pain and use of analgesics and years of poorer function,[57] there are increasing calls for screening for, and resolution of, mental health issues in order to achieve effective pain relief or control.[58] As meeting this need would create its own burden, given the paucity of mental health treatments available, it represents a further motivation impelling the search for alternatives.

Pain-specific psychological constructs

It is widely acknowledged in the pain medicine community that, in addition to psychological predispositions and vulnerabilities to developing chronic pain, there are psychological patterns which emerge in response to pain and then in turn shape the experience of pain and pain-related outcomes over time. Two of the most influential explanatory models which seek to describe and understand these processes are concerned with, respectively, the roles of catastrophizing and fear avoidance.

Catastrophizing

Catastrophizing describes an exaggerated negative orientation towards actual or anticipated pain experiences that involves: difficulty controlling pain-related thoughts; excessive focus (rumination) on pain sensations; magnification of the threat value of pain, including pain-related interpretations of ambiguous signals which interfere with other cognitive activities as well as physical tasks; a sense of being unable to cope with pain symptoms.[59] Catastrophizing is an instance, of course, of cognitive error in Beck's model of depression. Indeed, as a form of distorted cognition leading to negative emotional affect, catastrophizing is often barely distinguishable from a depressive cycle of behaviours and symptoms – helplessness, pessimism, rumination – and often correlates with the latter. A study of a large chronic pain patient sample found that catastrophizing was one of the most significant factors accounting for depression severity[60] and is known to have a negative impact on mental health, general health perception, social functioning and vitality.[61]

But while catastrophizing clearly overlaps with numerous other psychological processes, studies have shown that it is an independent contributor to the impact and experience of pain and has a 'unique and specific' influence on pain-related outcomes.[62] It is significantly associated, for example, with prolonged work absence,[63] risk for opioid misuse[64] and suicidal ideation.[65] Importantly, a higher level of catastrophizing has been shown to be a risk factor for the development of long-term pain, and for multiple negative sequelae of pain, including (in addition to those listed above) worsening physical disability and the intensification of pain sensitivity among patients. Studies have related catastrophizing, for example, to inflammatory responses to acute painful stimulation,[66] suggesting that catastrophizing sensitizes the nervous system to promote an amplification of pain transmission. Alongside a psychophysical increase in pain, catastrophizers experience reduced pain relief from both medication[67] and pain-relieving surgeries.[68] The vicious circle completes itself in findings which show that catastrophizing predicts more frequent seeking of medical care and higher consumption of pain-related drugs. It is strongly associated with heightened *craving* of opioids which in turn is one of the strongest determinants of opioid misuse.[69]

Catastrophizing often thus emerges as one of the most important predictors of the development of chronic pain. The combination of high pain catastrophizing and high depression severity at the onset of pain is consistently more likely to result in the worst outcomes.[70] Early intervention, before the pain becomes chronic, is deemed especially crucial for catastrophizers, since strongly held alarmist beliefs may be particularly potent in the early weeks of the condition. The indications are that early treatment changes in catastrophizing influence outcomes and recovery and, significantly, that psychosocial interventions (as we shall see) can be effective in this regard.

Fear avoidance

The Fear Avoidance model – a highly influential psychological account of the exacerbation or maintenance of pain – describes how pain-related fear, often interacting or interrelated with the cognitive and affective processes described above, sets in train its own vicious cyclical sequence of chronic disability. At the heart of the model is a person's belief about their pain.[71] If the pain is regarded as a temporary interruption or passing nuisance, then daily activity is usually resumed after a short interval. The problem begins when the person catastrophizes their pain as a signal of impending threat: that is to say, the pain is interpreted (contrary to the underlying biomedical pathology) as a sign of serious injury or illness over which the person has no control and which must necessarily lead to disability and can only be treated medically. This misinterpretation leads to a cascade effect in which an exaggerated fear of the pain extends to excessive fear of movement and activities which, it is presumed, could give rise to injury and pain, and thence to avoidance of these activities in order to elude the dangers perceived to accompany them.[72] Because avoidance rules out the opportunity to attune expectations to actual experiences and verify whether assumptions of impending danger are accurate or not, the tendency to overestimate future pain is itself exacerbated, and avoidant behaviour thus contributes to the self-perpetuating cycle of pain, catastrophizing and fear.[73] As avoidance amplifies fears, so heightened fear decreases the inclination to be physically active: reduced levels of physical activity lead to physical deconditioning or even disuse, which lowers the threshold at which pain is experienced.[74] All the while, vulnerability to emotional and psychological pain and suffering is exacerbated by the reluctance or inability to engage in valued pursuits or pastimes and by the inevitable social isolation which ensues.[75] This is a classic example of an evolutionary mode of preservation being turned against itself. Where avoidance makes sense in the short term, shielding the body from harm and allowing time to heal, in the case of chronic pain, the pain is no longer a signal of threat, rendering avoidance not only devoid of its protective function but ensuring its damaging potential for forging a route to acquired disability.[76]

Multiple studies show an association between fear avoidance behaviour and the experience of more intense pain, functional disability, poorer treatment outcomes and lower levels of return to work and suggest pain-related fear may influence the transition from acute to chronic pain.[77] Conversely, reductions in pain-related anxiety predict reduced distress, experience of pain and interference with daily activity, as well as improvements in functioning, clinical outcomes and the probability of return to work. The efficacy of targeted psychosocial treatments is perhaps partially explained by the fact that the fear avoidance model makes sense to pain sufferers themselves, insofar as it 'offers explanations that resonate with personal experience, and avoids punitive concepts such as secondary gain' (the idea that illness brings advantages – missing work, for example, or other commitments).[78]

While there is a general lack of definitive evidence for catastrophizing and fear avoidance as causal mechanistic influences on the trajectory of chronic pain, or as identifying universal pathways leading to pain-related disability, recent findings support the central importance of interactions among these overlapping factors. These processes contribute, in other words, to the 'cumulative risk load', which is regarded as key to individual pain trajectories. Needless to say, 'those with a higher cumulative risk load are more likely to develop prolonged pain and disability'.[79] One stark way of offering a rounded understanding of cumulative risk load, and how it shapes long-term pain-related outcomes, is by turning to the part played by trauma in the development of chronic pain.

Chronic pain and (childhood) trauma

The association between childhood abuse and serious (physical and mental) health problems in adulthood – both medically explained and unexplained – has become well established in recent decades. The evidence to show that maltreatment as a child predicts the later development of chronic pain is alarmingly and overwhelmingly strong. The presence of past trauma is associated with a two to threefold increase in the subsequent development of chronic pain and reports of abuse in childhood produce a 97 per cent increase in risk of experiencing a physical pain syndrome in adulthood.[80] Among patients with chronic pain in primary care settings, the prevalence of reported childhood physical or sexual abuse runs as high as 70 per cent.[81] Childhood abuse is associated with an abundance of physical complaints, and the degree of pain reported by abuse survivors in relation to these medical issues is consistently and significantly higher than the experience of pain reported by people with no abuse history.[82] Adult survivors of abuse, that is to say, have more pain-related health problems and more painful symptoms and the more severe the abuse, the more severe the pain.[83] The implications of these findings are formidable given the probability that children who experience one type of abuse are likely to be exposed to a cluster of related adversities, such as family conflict, parental absence, abandonment or divorce, and parental psychiatric disorder.[84] Sexual abuse is twice as common in women as in men, and a strong predictor of impairment of physical functioning in adult life, nearly doubling the chances of confinement to bed or limitation of usual activity.[85]

But what accounts for the significantly higher prevalence of *chronic* pain specifically among child abuse survivors? Some of the medical issues associated with a history of child abuse can be traced back to the physical injury or damage caused by the abusive treatment itself.[86] Poorer health outcomes can also be partly attributable to the higher likelihood that abuse survivors will engage in 'high-risk health behaviours'[87] (such as smoking, drug and alcohol abuse, overeating, non-safe sexual behaviour). Sometimes, moreover, it is the constellation of somatic symptoms which is bundled into specific diagnoses such as chronic pain or framed as medically unexplained somatic symptoms.[88] But the fact that the association of depression with a history of childhood abuse is even stronger than the latter's association with chronic pain has situated child abuse and associated psychological disorders as key causal factors in the development of chronic pain syndrome. Adults who experience abuse, neglect or serious family dysfunction as children are more likely to become depressed early in life, to experience recurrent depression and to be liable to major depressive disorder, as well as other types of psychiatric illness and psychological symptoms, such as anxiety, social phobia, eating disorders, and alcohol and drug dependence.[89] Again, the greater the range and severity of maltreatment experienced, the higher the probability of lifetime chronic or recurrent depression. Vulnerability to depressive symptoms in abuse survivors is exacerbated by multiple health complaints and frequent visits to medical and emergency care facilities (where abuse survivors often encounter negative patient-provider interactions) and a tendency towards low self-esteem, poor coping and interpersonal skills, and minimal social support.[90]

There are special reasons to infer that depression and chronic pain are particularly mutually maintaining, neurologically as well as psychologically, for abuse survivors. As we shall see in more detail in Chapter 3, a physiological consequence of early life trauma is enhanced sensitivity of the neurobiological systems which respond to stress. This results in overexposure to the stress hormone cortisol.[91] Too much cortisol in the body's circulation ('hypercortisolism') suppresses immune system response and increases the chance of illness.[92] Depression is likewise associated with dysregulation of cortisol and subsequent impaired immune functioning.[93] The neurochemical link to depression 'may render the individual less able to control pain or more vulnerable to pain owing to stress-induced pathophysiologic states like hypercortisolism'.[94] Neurochemical and psychological explanations thus converge or are mutually reciprocal in suggesting that chronic physical pain in this instance is an expression of chronic psychological pain.[95]

The psychiatric diagnosis which has been found most to strengthen the predictive relation between child abuse and the later development of chronic pain is the presence of Post-Traumatic Stress Disorder (PTSD). Resulting from exposure to a traumatic event, the key symptom of PTSD is the involuntary re-experiencing of the incident as well as hypervigilance in relation to stressors and consequent hypercortisolism. PTSD has been identified as a risk factor for chronic pain,[96] for the transition from acute to chronic pain,[97] and for elevated severity of pain and disability in abuse victims.[98] A thirty-year prospective study found there was a 'synergistic effect' whereby 'the combination of a history of child abuse and PTSD led to a marked increase in pain complaints'.[99] PTSD and pain do not simply co-occur and mutually maintain one another: one predicts the other, at the very least, as a marker of stress (and thus pain) vulnerability, and also insofar as PTSD hyperarousal has been associated with increased pain perception.[100] Moreover, the presence of current stressful life events has been found to more than double the effect of past physical or sexual abuse on health problems. Women with a history of abuse report more physical symptoms in response to daily stress than women with no abuse history.[101] Almost inevitably, given that those who have suffered neglect or maltreatment in childhood are more likely to become victims of abuse as adults,[102] one of the stressors frequently associated with physical symptoms and psychological distress is current abuse, especially domestic interpersonal.[103] 'The links between trauma and pain may summate cumulatively across the lifespan' such that 'the association of adult experienced trauma' (exposure to violence, for example) 'with deleterious pain-related outcomes' (such as PTSD) 'may reflect the cumulative effect of multiple historical traumas as well'.[104] '*As well*': past and present pain multiply in relation to one another and are experienced simultaneously. Cumulative risk load – not one thing after, but one thing on top of, another – is heavy indeed.

The chronic pain brain

In consideration of the multiplicity of factors determining the individual psychopathology of chronic pain, this section and the next turn, respectively, to neurobiological and social-environmental issues. The relation of this book's concerns with recent developments in neuroscience is the subject of Chapter 3, but I adumbrate here key new discoveries in respect of the neurobiology of chronic pain, which demonstrate that no one aspect of chronic pain is ever separable from another in the context of lived experience.

Brain imaging studies show that multiple neural systems are implicated in chronic pain. None of these are uniquely associated with pain. Rather, they are also involved in sensory, motor, cognitive and emotional functions, including memory and planning, anticipations of the probable outcomes (good or bad) of certain behaviours, evaluating what to expect of unknown conditions or unfamiliar circumstances and motivation towards or rank ordering of external stimuli.[105] Pain, then, entails a widely distributed and variably accessible neural network. It is not an inevitable consequence of 'noxious stimuli' – ones that threaten to damage the integrity of the body, such as injuring its tissue, for example. On the contrary, the neural systems which interpret the pain response are an intervolved mix of emotional, empathetic and anticipatory networks,[106] and, research suggests, can be accessed by non-sensory inputs (empathy for others' pain, social exclusion, hypnotically induced pain) to produce pain-like experiences.[107]

Nonetheless, neuroimaging has begun to identify features common to chronic pain sufferers which have key implications for understanding, and, as we shall see, for the treatment of the condition. One such feature is the discovery of alterations in structure, function and neurochemistry in the prefrontal cortex (PFC) of chronic pain sufferers when they are compared with healthy, pain-free controls.[108] Arriving late in evolutionary terms, yet undergoing dramatic expansion during mammalian development, the PFC, housed in the forehead, is regarded as centrally involved in the executive functions of the brain, the mental processes (insight, foresight, attentional focus and cognitive flexibility) that allow us to prioritize, problem-solve and self-regulate, and which are implicated more generally in personality, identity and meaningful action.[109] The PFC does not contain any primary sensory areas or react to stimulation directly. Rather, it controls or guides other brain activities, organizing, encoding, evaluating, verifying and monitoring material, including what is stored in long-term memory. As Steven Rose puts it in *The Twenty-First Century Brain*, this area 'is clearly *acting upon* information which has already received quite sophisticated analysis . . . processing inputs from multiple sensory systems and relating them to prior experience. Just as the brain as a whole is not a single organ but an accretion of less- and more-recently evolved structures . . . so too is the cortex'.[110] While integrating sensory inputs and linking them to motor outputs (muscular movements and behaviours) is a function of the entire brain, the sheer magnitude and extent of the PFC's connectivity give it a unique role in directing complex cognitive and emotional behaviours. The PFC figures in the majority of chronic pain-related imaging studies because it is the neurocircuit vital in regulating the perception and emotional-behavioural expression of pain in humans through reinterpretation, reappraisal – and tolerance of – adverse events.[111]

One compelling discovery of neuroscience in recent decades is a strong association between chronic pain and a decrease in grey matter volume and connectivity in the PFC.[112] The high concentration of neuronal cell bodies in grey matter and the latter's consequent essential role in information processing in the brain mean that any loss of density has implications for normal function in most aspects of human life – movement control, emotion regulation, memory retention. Unsurprisingly, consistent evidence across diverse chronic pain conditions of an alteration in grey matter density and connectivity, in the area of the brain whose multi-integrative and tightly interrelated structures play a critical role in emotional and cognitive processing in pain,[113] has enormously influenced the direction of chronic pain theory, research and treatment in recent years. There is strong interest in the degree to which these structural changes, which correlate significantly with the duration of the experience of chronic pain, are implicated in the transition from acute to chronic pain.[114] This is especially the case as there is growing (though inconclusive) evidence that these changes in brain structure are a consequence (and a potentially reversible one) rather than a cause.[115]

A further related discovery prompted by the neuroimaging revolution is that reduced neural connectivity in people living with chronic pain can hardwire circuit pathways between brain areas associated with negative emotions and pain perception. While the science underlying these conclusions is complex and the intricacies impossible to represent judiciously outside of a neuroscientific journal paper, the implications for the chronic pain sufferer are highly intuitive. Noting heightened patterns of activity in regions already tightly interconnected to the PFC and associated with threat detection as well as emotion and memory processing, researchers have hypothesized that chronic pain engages this emotional and memory-processing region of the brain into a state of continued negative emotions. The memory traces accumulated since the onset of pain – as well as those prior to it – continue to be stored as long as the pain carries on, and are reinforced by further sensory inputs that perpetuate the state. The specific individual signature of this reorganization of brain circuitry may be critical in the transition from acute to chronic pain, on the one hand (with all the psychological costs which can result) or, on the other hand, in the ceasing of pain and the return to life as usual.[116] Chronic pain, say the authors of this study, 'is a persistence of the memory of pain and/or the inability to extinguish the memory of pain evoked by an initial inciting injury'. Pain's close relationship with memory is part of its survival value: once bitten, twice shy as the old adage says. But such 'fear conditioning' (to use a Pavlovian or behavioural term) is also what underlies phobias, panic attacks and PTSD. The 'novel hypothesis' advanced by these researchers is 'that chronic pain is a state of continuous learning, in which aversive emotional associations are continuously made with incidental events, simply due to the persistent presence of pain':

> A concrete example might further clarify this idea: A person with chronic pain enters his/her bedroom. Depending on the intensity of the pain at that moment, the person establishes a negative association with the bedroom (place conditioned avoidance), and the stronger the pain the longer lasting will be the memory of this negative association. Given that the person has pain all the time, whenever he/she re-enters the bedroom, the negative association is reinforced, and thus there is no chance for extinction (erasing the negative association) by exposure to the space in the absence of pain. Of course, the person is rationally aware that the bedroom is not the source of the pain but his/her emotional system continues to provide contradictory cues. We propose that living with this conundrum and the effort of disentangling its associations underlies at least some of the suffering of chronic pain, and comprises an important component of the cortical negative emotional impact of neuropathic pain.[117]

Though the authors do not discount the possibility of genetic predisposition to cortical reorganization and learnt associations that reinforce and sustain pain, the logic of this example is that the processes that harden into a chronic pain state are to some degree reversible, and are connected to emotional disentangling – rewiring or reset – that is simultaneously behavioural, psychological and neural. There is a nexus of entry points, that is to say, for this task of healing reorganization.

Social and environmental influences on chronic pain

Pain's demographic is, in certain ways, less complex – or at least more stark – than its biopsychology, though the interpenetration of the two is often varied and tangled and the same affective patterns often appear.

Recent research suggests that the occurrence of chronic pain rises with advancing age,[118] for the logical reason that older people have had more exposure both to the types of injury and stimuli that can trigger chronic pain as well as to the 'cumulative risk load' of multi-morbidity.[119] Chronic pain is by no means age-limited, however, as we have begun to see. In a study involving forty-two countries, over 20 per cent of young people reported experiencing some form of chronic pain and the condition appears to affect up to 30 per cent of people aged 18–39.[120] A large Europe-wide study found that the 41–60 age group suffered more than people either younger or older.[121] The study also affirmed the virtually universal finding that chronic pain is more prevalent among women than men. Women experience higher pain intensity and pain-related disability than men.[122] This gender-specific difference has been variously accounted for by sex-specific hormones or genes, lower pain thresholds and 'maladaptive coping strategies'.[123] Amid the near-ubiquitous call for further research in this area, there is recognition of the need to take into account, for example, greater female vulnerability to interpersonal violence and the psychological repercussions which are risk factors for long-term pain.[124]

What is true of both men and women, of all ages, is that behaviours already known to affect health adversely make chronic pain worse. Smoking is a causal factor in conditions closely associated with the onset of chronic pain,[125] and people affected by chronic pain are more likely to smoke more heavily and to struggle to give up the habit.[126] Alcohol is commonly used to alleviate pain. Overuse leads to resistance to alcohol's analgesic effects, while alcohol withdrawal symptoms increase pain sensitivity; both lead to escalating use at higher doses to compensate, and increased dependency.[127] Obesity heightens chronic pain by putting strain on weight-bearing joints and reducing physical activity, with the plethora of health and psychosocial issues we have already seen this to create.[128] Many of these 'lifestyle choices' are associated with socio-economic demographics which are themselves found to be a risk factor for, or to coincide with, the prevalence of chronic pain. The occurrence of chronic pain has been reliably shown to relate inversely to socio-economic status. A recent UK study found, firstly, that the prevalence of chronic pain among people earning below £18,000 per annum was 52.5 per cent, as compared with 33.5 per cent among those earning above £100,000 per annum; and, secondly, that while chronic pain affected 39.8 per cent of people in paid employment and 42.4 per cent of people in voluntary or unpaid work, it affected 78.9 per cent of people who were unemployed.[129] It is not merely that there is a higher incidence of chronic pain among people from low-income groups, who are disadvantaged educationally and environmentally, than among their better-housed, well-educated, more affluent fellow citizens; the pain they suffer is more severe and the level of pain-related disability they experience is more extreme. Inequality and pain are mutually exacerbating: people in low-income groups are more susceptible to pain and more liable to unemployment because of their pain. Job loss or change may cause financial strains as well as a sense of loss of purpose. These instabilities can affect marital, family and social relationships, leading to loneliness, a low sense of self-worth and mood (and sleep) disturbances.[130] This is not the first time this chapter has rounded this circle, and I trace its contours again here to emphasize its apparent ineluctability wherever we seek to understand the determinants of chronic pain.

For ethnic groups, this cycle tightens even further. Extensive evidence has accumulated since the 1990s, mostly, though not exclusively, from the United States, that 'the burden of pain is unequal across racial and ethnic groups'.[131] The reasons for these disparities in experience, management and treatment of pain are complex and variable across ethnicities and cultures,[132] but there are clear patterns suggesting consistent under-treatment of pain among non-white populations. Language barriers, lack of easy access to interpreters and cultural differences in styles of communication affect not only the quality of interaction between the patient and healthcare professional, including the efficacy of the questioning around symptoms, expression of empathic concern and the sense of collaborative decision-making. It also has an impact on pain sufferers' knowledge of available treatments, general health literacy and health outcomes given that patients' capacity to adhere to pain treatment and management programmes is impaired by these factors.[133]

Unconscious bias and discrimination on the part of caregivers are perhaps the most important factors explaining disparities in treatment.[134] In addition to the well-documented health inequalities experienced by pain sufferers from ethnic minorities, they are more likely to have the severity of their pain underestimated. One study carried out in the United States found that, while Black patients reported more intense pain and worse disability than their white counterparts, they were rated as having less pain and received fewer radiographs and advanced imaging studies, as well as less surgery and hospitalization.[135] Ethnic minority pain patients are less likely to receive comprehensive diagnoses and appropriate and specialized treatment,[136] have longer wait times and are less likely to have their pain needs met in both emergency and hospice care.[137] Implicit bias manifests itself particularly in respect of pharmacological treatments. A large US survey found that white people were more likely to endanger themselves with drugs and that the overall rate of drug-related deaths was highest among non-Hispanic white people. African-Americans and Hispanics were found to be more afraid than non-Hispanic whites of opioid addiction and less likely to misuse prescription opioids. Nonetheless, African-American and Hispanic patients were less likely than white people to receive medication as part of their pain management regime and received lower doses based on the misconception that Black and Hispanic patients should have less access to drugs because they are at greater risk than white patients of abusing them.[138]

The discriminatory practices must be understood in the context of three considerations. Firstly, the higher reported incidence of pain in non-white people. In one large population study in the United States, 27 per cent of African-Americans and 28 per cent of Hispanics over fifty years old reported experiencing severe pain most of the time, as compared with 17 per cent of white people in the same age category.[139] Secondly, the danger of under-treating pain, which, uncontrolled, as we have seen, reduces mobility, strength and increases susceptibility to psychological illnesses.[140] Thirdly, the possibility that perceived bias is related to the experience of pain.[141] Perceived discrimination has been found to be associated with more bodily pain among African-, Chinese-, and Hispanic-Americans.[142] Around 50 per cent of Hispanic people and 70 per cent of Black people in the United States report experiencing unfair treatment because of their ethnicity. Discrimination is associated with increased psychological distress[143] which, as we have seen, is related to the development of chronic pain. Thus, as well as experiencing more difficulty than their white counterparts in persuading health care providers of the severity of their pain, non-white sufferers believe that health professionals do not understand their pain, do not believe them when they say they are in pain and do not care about their pain.[144] Greater hopelessness produces worse pain management outcomes and worsened expectations of the efficacy of the treatment prescribed.

In fact, for pain sufferers in general, the degree of perceived caring by and from others is another critical aspect of the social environment in its power to shape pain experience, management and health outcomes. The quality, nature and degree of interpersonal support contribute significantly to either improved functioning or increased pain-related disability. It is worth recalling at this point how much long-term chronic pain affects ordinary, day-to-day, domestic life and for how long. One European survey showed that one-third of people with chronic pain are in severe pain; roughly half are in constant pain. Most have had pain for at least two years and one-fifth for twenty years or longer. Two-thirds of people were less able to sleep because of their pain, half found household chores difficult, two-fifths experienced problems with sexual relations and one-fifth felt inadequate as a spouse or partner.[145] As a sense of helplessness is often compounded by the distrust, scepticism and disbelief pain sufferers frequently encounter from doctors, colleagues, friends and family, it is not surprising that the attitude of significant others can be crucial in determining the degree to which the vicious circles chronic pain generates – inactivity begets depression which begets further inactivity – can be broken. As an encouraging partner might help alleviate avoidant fear, for example, so low levels of support in the workplace, including the need to confront the vagaries of social or occupational compensation schemes, can exacerbate depression and disability.[146]

These negative attitudes are engendered in part, as we have seen, by the 'invisible' nature of chronic pain – the lack of obvious physical cause for the experience of severe pain and the impairments to ordinary living which it entails. Chronic pain sufferers commonly face the dead end of there being no medical foundation for their pain, no obvious means of alleviation and responses from the medical establishment which create self-doubt and distrust of health carers. In the Europe-wide study cited above, 40 per cent reported that their pain was not managed well, was overlooked or not considered a problem.[147] A consequence of this experience with health providers, ironically, is that 'commonly chronic pain sufferers become high users of the medical system in search of validation for their experiences, an explanation for their pain, palliative treatment, and even a cure'.[148] Herewith, another entirely non-virtuous circle. This relationship with the care system is the more alarming given that studies demonstrate that creating and sustaining a sound and effective therapeutic relationship or 'alliance'[149] stimulates patient expectations that treatment will help and is a crucial foundation for the success of the pain-improving effects of myriad interventions.

Psychosocial treatments

Cognitive behavioural therapy (CBT)

This brings me to the role of interpersonal therapy in clinical contexts in relation to chronic pain. While most treatment plans and programmes blend medical, psychological, vocational, educational and alternative treatment techniques,[150] unsurprisingly, in view of the overwhelming evidence for social and psychological influences on the condition, as well as the dubious efficacy and outright dangers of pharmacological and surgical interventions, current recommendations for best practice in the treatment of chronic pain emphasize 'outcomes that focus on improvements in quality of life' and 'safer and less invasive treatments'.[151] The most widely researched and practised psychological intervention is CBT, which, with a foundation in both ancient philosophy[152] and classic (Skinnerian) behaviourist principles, developed in part out of the success of cognitive therapies for depression pioneered by Beck and others in the 1970s. Cognitive therapy 'emphasised the critical meditational role played by idiosyncratic interpretations of events in determining a person's emotional and behavioural responses to event', and targeted 'dysfunctional thinking' and negative 'underlying schema and modes of information processing'.[153] Given the marked overlap between pain and depression, components of Beck's therapy were adapted to the treatment of chronic pain. CBT, as we shall see in Part II, was the comparator intervention for our study of literary reading, both because it represented an aspect of treatment as usual and because this standard psychosocial therapy offered the closest available and appropriate non-pharmacological paradigm to the power of literary reading to influence chronic pain.

CBT's objectives in relation to chronic pain are essentially threefold. Firstly, 'to help patients change their view of their problem from overwhelming to manageable' in order that 'what could be perceived as a hopeless condition can be reframed as difficult yet [one] over which they can exercise some control'. This includes 'helping patients to realise that short-term increases in pain do not necessarily signal tissue damage or progressing pathology'. Secondly, to convince patients of the 'need to be actively involved in their treatment and rehabilitation'. Thirdly, 'to teach patients to monitor maladaptive thoughts and substitute more realistic, functional thoughts'. Demonstrating 'how and when to attack these negative thoughts and when to substitute more realistic thoughts and adaptive management techniques for chronic pain is an important component of cognitive restructuring'.[154] CBT for chronic pain, delivered to individuals or in groups, typically involves structured steps and sub-goals aimed at directly assessing thoughts associated with pain, identifying behaviour that is contingent on pain and altering psychological processes, such as catastrophizing or pain-related fear, which, as we have seen, contribute to pain, distress and disability. Evidence from CBT studies not only indicates that changes in catastrophizing precede changes in clinical pain,[155] but that CBT produces substantial reductions in catastrophizing even among patients whose chronic pain has lasted for decades.[156] The treatment's catastrophizing-reducing effects, moreover, may last for months or years.[157] This is an especially important consideration given that, as mentioned earlier, much of the variability in treatment benefit and outcomes can be accounted for by early treatment changes in catastrophizing. Moreover, such benefits of CBT are most directly analogous, as will become apparent in Part II, to the potential of literary reading to offer powerful alternative perspectives on pain and on the life within which it is suffered.

While the evidence base for the effectiveness of chronic pain is currently larger and stronger for CBT than for other psychological interventions, and, significantly, on a par with pharmacological and physical treatments, proving definitively the efficacy of CBT by the commonest scientific method (the Randomized Controlled Trial) has nevertheless proved problematic. Although 'CBT for pain has been widely implemented as a standard treatment for pain and constitutes the current "gold standard" for psychological intervention for pain',[158] the intervention is not itself *standardized*. The term CBT covers widely varying strategies, which may be more or less embedded in comprehensive pain management programmes,[159] and which differ in mode (individual or group therapy), duration (a one-time occurrence, or commitment to a – usually short, time-limited – programme) and method. The latter can include, for example: psychoeducation about pain, behaviour and mood; formulation and repetition of positive self-statements or self-instruction; gradual exposure to feared situations and/or activities; strategies for relaxation and problem-solving; distraction techniques; positive event scheduling and goal-setting; and means of enhancing social support.[160] The quality of the treatment received is also highly variable. Unlike pharmacological treatments, psychological treatments are entirely manufactured by therapists at the point of delivery. Treatments are dynamic, constructed 'in the moment' and subject to the influence of context, including the group setting or individual patient. The heterogeneity of the model and its quality of delivery are compounded, according to one review of the scientific evidence, by under-theorized models of how CBT produces change, by the sheer complexity and multiplicity of health issues that go under the name of chronic pain and by the consequent diversity of participants and of the treatments they are receiving.

> Examination of what we think is feasible as the outcome of psychological treatment is appropriate: is it mere palliation, in which case effects will be small, or do we expect to move people who are stuck in trying to solve the unsolvable problem of pain to address instead the solvable problem of living more satisfactorily with chronic pain and starting to do so? Or to put it another way, do we believe that we effectively enable patients to manage the interruption of pain and to reduce its interference with their lives, and thereby to repair damaged identities.[161]

This question of what should be 'treated' where chronic pain is concerned, and how CBT and other psychosocial interventions are best employed in this respect, is one which recurs across this book and one to which I return in Part III and the Afterword. Certainly, the protean nature of such models – where diverse shapes and forms and contextual applications of the therapy are more often the rule than the exception – has substantial potential advantages, whatever the obstacles thereby presented to scientific study even of those very benefits. Psychosocial interventions can be readily combined with other treatments and interventions, as well as modified for specific circumstances and individual needs. Significantly, the review cited above recommends fewer large-scale Randomized Controlled Trials and a focus instead on, for example, 'examining individual data for response trajectories'.[162] This connects directly with a key axiom of Engel's biopsychosocial model of health, which largely underwrites the clinical understanding and approach to chronic pain that I have outlined in this chapter: 'In scientific work the investigator is generally obliged to select one system level on which to concentrate, or at least at which to begin, his efforts. For the physician, that system level is always *person*, i.e. a patient.'[163]

Access to psychological therapies and social prescribing

The relation of physician to patient in respect of making decisions on healthcare plans has taken on a new dimension with the advent of self-referral and social prescribing schemes in the UK over the past two decades. As this is the care context within which both CBT and the Shared Reading model with which it is compared in Part II loosely operate, and within which Shared Reading's future as a 'treatment' option is likely to be situated, a critical understanding of the state of play is valuable and I will return to it in my conclusion also.

Self-referral has become a routine aspect of mental health care as part of NHS schemes such as England's 'Improving Access to Psychological Therapies' (IAPT). Begun in 2008, the scheme sought to provide large-scale support for common mental health problems (mild to moderate anxiety and depression) at a time of rising demand and pressure on GPs, as well as encouraging parity of care and resource allocation between mental and physical health conditions. Self-referral can offer more flexibility than GP surgery hours, avoid stigma and initiate access to alternatives to pharmacological treatment. While such strategies demonstrate a commitment to ensuring that (destigmatized and de-medicalized) mental health provision is available to everyone who needs it, there is evidence that self-referral is a barrier to seeking psychological therapies, particularly among low-income groups. In their study of doctor-patient interactions around IAPT, Felicity Thomas et al. found that there was a 'disconnect' between GPs' representation of self-referral as 'straightforward', and patients' sense of the challenge of engaging with others when feeling low or distressed. There was an expressed need for an 'extra push' to 'take the first step to help themselves' or someone 'to open a door for you'. For low-income patients, the 'enormity' of self-referral was exacerbated by the day-to-day experience of having to 'fight' for welfare services, under which circumstances the effort of accessing IAPT seemed an overwhelming process and another instance of being underserving or unentitled. While those for whom booking and attending the GP appointment had taken courage felt 'fobbed off' by the IAPT self-referral leaflet, those (rare) patients who had a GP referral felt their health concerns were being validated by a '"legitimate" source of authority'. Thus, where GPs in the study tended to welcome and encourage self-referral as an exercise of autonomous choice and self-agency, those charged with the task of 'helping themselves' and 'taking ownership' of the treatment process felt their health concerns to be delegitimized and dismissed which increased despondency and alienation. Moreover, the efficacy of self-referral is questionable. Thomas's study found that 40 per cent of those who received a self-referral recommendation did not follow through with it, and that those who did encountered a range of frustrations, including wait times between stages of support.[164] This finding is not apparently contradicted by official figures. A 2019 blog by one of the founders of IAPT, celebrating ten years of the programme, stated that the service was reaching over 1,000,000 people each year, with 'approximately half undertaking a course of therapy', and others 'receiving an assessment, advice and signposting to services'. With the outcomes thus vague and variable and the blog's prediction that 'the number of people with anxiety disorders or depression who can access help each year through IAPT [will] reach 1.9 million by 2024', the current reliance on self-referral to psychological therapies may be unprecedented, and thus its hidden gaps and insufficiencies in support for mental health increasing accordingly.[165]

These issues are brought into still sharper focus when the relatively unregulated and unmonitored practice of social prescribing is concerned. As Helen Chatterjee explains, social prescribing is 'an innovative approach to public health, as it advocates the use of voluntary and third sector organisations and creates referral pathways so that primary care patients with non-clinical needs can be directed to these sources of community intervention'.[166] As with IAPT, the growth of social prescribing has been motivated both by a need to expand options available to GPs – who are increasingly under-resourced in the face of a mental health crisis caused by that same climate of austerity – and by influential government publications, such as the Marmot review into health inequalities in England (2010), which focused on the social determinants of disparities in health outcomes across the population and emphasized the importance of sustainable and empowered individuals and communities in ill health prevention.[167] These are the key areas which, as Chatterjee points out, social prescribing has historically addressed. Three of the most established models – Arts on Prescription (creative and participatory workshops in dance, drama, music, painting and poetry), Books on Prescription (referral to self-help books using CBT principles) and Exercise on Prescription (referring patients to supported exercise programmes) – offer 'sources of support . . . for people with social, emotional, or practical needs, . . . considered vulnerable or at risk . . . living with long-term health conditions [or] in social isolation'.[168] The predominant model is for people to be connected by health professionals to a Link Worker who, with local knowledge, identifies appropriate community activities. There is a high degree of local variation in types of social prescribing, which, on the one hand, has the advantage of providing 'a wide range of opportunities to people across all age groups, different ability levels, and various physical and mental health needs, and [potentially] a more comprehensive approach than other schemes'. Studies have demonstrated the value of participation in terms of enhanced self-expression, self-esteem, sense of purpose, quality of life and stress reduction.[169] On the other hand, says a 2019 editorial in the *British Journal of General Practice*, such heterogeneity is a 'function of social prescribing being the demand-driven formalisation of referrals to existing community services and organisations', which means that it 'has proliferated without a concomitant evidence base'.[170] The limited resources of local organizations for evaluation of their services, the difficulty of generalizing from local context-bound models and the multiple components and variables of social prescription are all factors that make it inimical to standard, 'robust' health research design, which anyway may not capture some of the subtle benefits of, for example, arts and creative activity.[171] For some critics of social prescribing, the issues are much more fundamental still. Rob Poole and Peter Huxley, who describe themselves as belonging to a generation of mental health professionals committed to community care ('We worked in large mental hospitals, and we have no nostalgia for them'), have recently argued that the tendency to present social prescribing as an appropriate response to health issues with social determinants means that 'an ill-defined intervention' is inappropriately 'framed as a "solution" to complex problems' caused by prolonged underfunding of social infrastructures and the latter's effect on the poorest sectors of the population. Not only does this 'obscure any useful role [social prescribing] might have' (in providing alternatives for health practitioners 'who are uncomfortable with medicating the effects of adversity', for example). More problematic still, it 'constrain[s] the role of general practitioners to signposting' and thereby effectively betrays Engels's biopsychosocial model of health. 'A care process that has sequestrated the social from the medical and psychological is entirely inimical [to] a strong commitment to caring for people [by] taking their psychological and social contexts as seriously as biological aspects of their ill health.'[172] Thomas, too, calls for, and has sought to implement, a practice of 'working out which [treatments] make sense to the patient based on a shared biopsychosocial model, . . . providing time for people to think and discuss their options'.[173] Building on her research on the over-representation of pharmacological treatments in areas of deprivation, Thomas has developed a training resource for GPs working with people suffering from poverty-related distress, encouraging '"micro-therapeutic" practices to build trust, identify strengths and discuss alternatives to antidepressants'.[174] These considerations are deeply serious ones in relation to a condition as complex as chronic pain, as we have seen, and need to be carefully weighed against recent evidence that there might be some advantage to *non-medical* referral routes for social prescribing. 'Sign-posting' via health practitioners (occupational therapists and hospital discharge teams as well as GPs) is 'not equitable', this research suggests, and 'could even be disproportionately reaching people who are *less* disadvantaged', while 'those who are under 16, male, and those from non-white backgrounds [are] less likely to be offered Social Prescribing'. In addressing the general urgent need for resources and infrastructure (given a shortage of community activities, the relative underutilization of the latter once contact with a link worker has been made, and the gaps in evidence of effectiveness), strategic planning 'should prioritise' referral routes which are non-medical (via voluntary organizations, housing associations, for example) to ensure that 'individuals from more deprived areas, younger adults, men, and ethnic minority groups [are] reached more equitably'.[175]

I return, of necessity, to these grave and knotty issues in the Afterword in final consideration of the place of Shared Reading within the current (complex and contentious) context of UK healthcare provision. I do so when the reader will have witnessed first-hand (from Part II) that what Shared Reading becomes in this context's discourses – a health intervention, or a social care tool – can seem far removed from what, essentially, it is. This is a further tension of 'arts' prescribing in particular, perhaps, and one which adds further complication to the issue of standardization of provision and 'quality assessment'.

I close this chapter now, however, with evidence which hints at a dimension that is sometimes missing (at least in application) even from Engel's comprehensive vision of health and which bears directly on the concerns of the next chapter. Certainly, what has been neglected in Randomized Controlled Trials of psychosocial interventions is the determining role of a key intrapersonal component: *belief* in the treatment's appropriateness and efficacy and consequent motivation to derive benefit from it. Among the 'individual characteristics' that lead to 'increased receptiveness' to CBT, for example, 'beliefs about treatment credibility and expectancy [are] both strongly associated with the outcome of CBT'.[176] Despite the acknowledged strength of the influence of belief, this dimension occupies little more than a footnote across the extensive research on psychosocial treatments in chronic pain. Herein lies my rationale and motivation for placing this clinical picture alongside a historical and enlarged therapeutic context for understanding chronic pain in the coming chapters. The intention is to point up, that is to say, how orientations towards chronic pain from distinct disciplines and knowledge bases have long pointed, implicitly, in a common direction.

2

Pain and meaning

Over the past half-century, pain, as a concept or construct as much as an experience, has enjoyed considerable attention outside of clinical contexts. Pain's place in the history of knowledge, culture and mind has exercised scholars from a range of disciplines and theoretical or ideological standpoints. In this chapter, I bring into dialogue with the clinical picture outlined in the previous section some of these multiple discourses and perspectives. The intention is not to undertake the (impossible) task of offering a comprehensive overview, but to map out common areas of enquiry and fruitful points of (often hitherto unseen or unacknowledged) connection or contact. The primary interest of the considerable and demonstrable overlap which emerges from this interchange of ideas is its value in laying a foundation for my focus in Part II on the contemporary uses of the culturally ancient practice of reading literature for people living with pain in the here and now.

Meaning

Across the medical and non-medical disciplines invoked by pain – which embrace anthropology, sociology and the arts, as well as history, philosophy and theology – there is a remarkable consensus that, as David B. Morris puts it in *The Culture of Pain*, 'Pain is almost always the occasion of an encounter with meaning. . . . We experience pain only and entirely as we interpret it'.[1] This is by no means of interest to theoretical hermeneutics only or primarily: on the contrary, it is at the centre of the pain experience. 'Our particular sensitivity to pain, and the anxiety that attends it, is not simply a matter of genetics, physiology and circumstance, vitally important as these are: the way we *interpret* our pain is all important for the mode of our suffering it.'[2] The established orthodoxy of this assumption is implicit in the psychological approaches to pain summarized in the previous section – in the attention to attributional style, to take one example – as well as in the emphasis on cognitive ('mind over matter') treatments such as CBT. Indeed, this orientation is explicit in Psychology in the development (for example) of an assessment instrument, the 'Pain Solutions Questionnaire', which incorporates a five-point scale examining the 'meaningfulness of life despite pain': higher scores on this scale (indicating a stronger sense of meaningfulness) were strongly correlated with lower scores on scales assessing attention to pain, catastrophizing, distress and pain-related disability.[3] The conclusion that the experience of meaning and the experience of pain go hand in hand is so ubiquitous in cross-disciplinary scholarship on pain because the phenomenon is itself apparently universal, occurring transculturally and transhistorically.

In historical surveys of pain, religious interpretations of the pain experience are one of the most prevalent and robust, even as they are often positioned as occupying a specific, and now outmoded, place in history. For pre-twentieth-century Western cultures steeped in Christian theology, pain had purposes, retributive or redemptive. Pain was a divinely appointed gift sent variously to chasten the sinner, purge corruption, change wayward habits, teach submission and instruct the sufferer in the path of righteousness, as well as preparing for a better life beyond the grave. In her study of the representation of pain in nineteenth-century culture – in which pain was common, severe and often cruel – Lucy Bending cites the influential Evangelical clergyman, J. C. Ryle, as representative of a tradition that interpreted pain theologically. The cause of the cholera outbreak of the 1860s was not, according to Ryle, '"bad drainage, bad water, want of cleanliness, want of sufficient food"' but '"The Hand of the Lord!" working on earth: a divine policy for bringing man's actions into line with God's will'. 'Christianity's peculiar power where physical pain is concerned lies, Ryle suggests, in the fact that The Hand of the Lord that inflicts such chastising pain is also "The hand that was nailed to the cross of Calvary."'[4] As Bending goes on to show, such readings of pain, firmly tied as they were to a belief in the literal truth of the Bible, were hard to sustain as the century progressed. The Christian justification of pain that had been accepted for centuries now faced three formidable and concurrent challenges. Firstly, from Broad Church liberalism, for which pain posed both a theological problem (insofar as it came to be regarded as an expression not of divine justice but of God's injustice), and an ethical one (as the moral rationalizations of pain seemed to fly in the face of a Christian duty to alleviate suffering). Secondly, from Darwinian theory, which gave grounds for understanding pain as a function and consequence of evolutionary development (both as a warning of danger and as a consequence of the gradual human transition from quadruped to biped). Thirdly, from advances in medical knowledge, above all the advent of anaesthetics. Chloroform undermined the characterization of pain both as a '*natural* phenomenon'[5] and 'as a spiritual good'.[6]

Cultural historians are understandably sceptical of the value of religious justifications of pain, which covertly or otherwise invited or validated oppressive practices and behaviours, and indeed suffering itself. 'Sacrifice, renunciation, expiation, purification, catharsis, and salvation are practised within an evaluative framework in which personal disposition is imposed upon mere physiology in such a way that it is not only possible to extract positive consequences from bodily torments, it is also possible to develop the idea that redemption or liberation depends on the mortification of the flesh.'[7] But as Joanna Bourke points out in *The Story of Pain*, religious narrative and language – unlike its (increasingly medicalized) secular counterpart – was 'rich' and 'restorative, not destructive'.[8] Moreover, its influence was not merely dogmatic and prescriptive, but profoundly personal and emotional. Bourke cites the instance of nineteenth-century Methodist, Joseph Townend, who, born into poverty in Northern England and almost mortally injured in infancy, underwent excruciatingly painful surgery in adulthood (without the aid of anaesthetic or analgesic) as a result of an accident in a textile factory. In the weeks that followed, he wept, read the Scriptures, sang hymns and, in his autobiography written a decade later, credited the period of suffering with returning him 'entirely [to] the Lord'. As Bourke says: the 'meanings he gave to his suffering had profound effects on the ways he experienced the agonizing sensations. . . . For the pious Townend, physical and spiritual anguish were inseparable'.[9]

Studies involving modern-day chronic pain patients suggest that, notwithstanding the historical trajectory traced by Dend-ing's thesis and indicated in Bourke's subtitle ('From Prayer to Painkillers'), there is some continuity between the experience of Townend, whose 'corporeal sensations were profoundly affected by his [religious] interpretation of what was happening to him',[10] and that of contemporary sufferers. In the last quarter of the twentieth century, researchers in social psychology in the United States found religious interpretation of pain and suffering to be common, and appraisal of serious instances as a reflection of God's will, more common than any other.[11] This is consistent with findings from early this century onwards of a tendency to seek spiritual support during times of illness and to pray for health-related concerns.[12] Though this area is still relatively neglected in chronic pain studies and pain medicine, the empirical evidence that exists, derived from different national and cultural populations, points towards religious belief as an influence on the experience of pain. A nationally representative study carried out in Canada concluded that 'Religion, as measured by worship frequency together with importance of spiritual values, is associated with lower levels of chronic pain and fatigue syndromes [and] better psychological well-being in the population with chronic pain and fatigue'.[13] Research undertaken in Germany found that 'utilization of spirituality/religiosity goes far beyond fatalistic acceptance, but can be regarded as an active coping process . . . in adjustment to chronic pain'.[14] A study involving highly devout Protestants in Denmark showed that prayer reduced subjective ratings of pain intensity and unpleasantness for religious participants;[15] and research among a multicultural population of older people in the Northern England (comprising Christians, Hindus, Sikhs, Jews and Muslims) found that faith provided not only a thought system to appraise the meaning and purpose of pain, but pain management strategies that were embedded directly in their religious beliefs (in prayer, religious texts and use of herbal preparations) or indirectly derived from the support received through the religious community.[16]

The significant interest in the first two decades of this century in the role of religion in chronic pain management owes something, no doubt, to the relative failure of pharmacological and surgical interventions in relation to chronic pain and the emphasis on holistic approaches to the condition. As the medical solutions that ousted religious ones a century or so ago have been found wanting, both older religious practices and their modern developments, derivatives or reinventions have gained currency once more. Bourke's chapter on pain and religion begins and ends with the compelling case of how Townend's very 'way of conceiving pain was inextricably related to his entire being-in-the-world', insofar as his bodily suffering 'was inextricably entangled with his upbringing as a Methodist [and] his spiritual beliefs'.[17] Amid the Western trend towards secularization and medicalization of suffering over the past two centuries, the kind of religious framework that supported Townend not only appears to remain relevant. Such religious conceptions of the lived experience of pain perhaps offer an ultimate example of how the experience of pain is always bound up with one's 'entire being-in-the-world'. In other words, one's way of being in the world and one's way of being in pain are never separable.

Total pain

I want to test this proposition in relation to the work of two (twentieth and twenty-first century) women (one English, one American) who are especially well positioned to offer an insider view of the relation of pain and meaning (including religious meaning) in modern secular times.

The first of these is Cicely Saunders, now universally accredited with founding the modern hospice movement and its grounding philosophy. Saunders was concerned exclusively with the care of the dying; but this pain is, by definition, incurably chronic, and its psychopathology, as Saunders herself pointed out, virtually indistinguishable from that of chronic pain as defined in Chapter 1. 'Although the terminal period of persistent malignant disease is often brief compared with some forms of chronic disease, its course (and its treatment) frequently delivers a series of blows, each destroying some part of the patient's capacity for normal and independent living.'[18] Her writings and insights thus have application and resonance beyond palliative care. Indeed, the current interest in 'the biopsychospiritual approach' – as the call for recognition of the role of religion and spirituality in pain care and medicine has become known – has largely been inspired by Saunders's pioneering work.[19]

Saunders came to her role as a physician in midlife. She read Philosophy, Politics and Economics at Oxford, and, when her studies were interrupted by the Second World War ('[I] had to give it up because it didn't seem the right place to be during wartime'[20]), she trained and worked as a nurse at St Thomas's Hospital, London, 'in the absence of nearly all our modern pharmacology'.[21] Her most recent biographer, David Clark, recounts how, in later life, she recalled with relish an earlier biographer's description of how she took to her first profession: 'like a book finding its right place on the shelf'. But 'in truth', as Clark goes on to say, 'this was a moment of transformational change'. A young woman brought up in middle-class affluence and educated at an elite school and university was entering a 'more visceral world . . . a place of death and suffering, and an environment of endless physical labour coupled with the constant personal and psychological demands of giving nursing care in extreme circumstances'.[22] As a result of this prolonged and arduous work, Saunders put out a spinal disc and was forced to give up nursing at the end of three years. She returned to Oxford to complete her degree, and (with a practical care-related profession now in view), also took a diploma in Public and Social Administration, fitting two years of studies into one ('her back . . . by now so painful that she did most of her reading laying down'[23]). During this time, she underwent a period of religious seeking and conversion under the several influences of the intellectually and socially engaged Christianity she encountered both in contemporary Oxford luminaries, such as C. S. Lewis, and in her extensive reading in the Evangelical Christian movement. Within weeks of her full conversion, she commenced her training as a medical social worker (known as a 'Lady Almoner' until 1964, reflecting the origin of the profession in Victorian charity and alms-giving[24]) in London terminal-care homes. Her experience of working 'among patients and families devastated by unrelieved pain in terminal cancer' confirmed Saunders in her vocation (and religious calling) of caring for the dying. With the nursing profession closed to her, she took the advice of a senior and distinguished surgeon at St Thomas's: 'Go and read medicine. It's the doctors who desert the dying and there's so much to be learned about pain.' Saunders undertook medical training 'during the pharmacological explosion of the 1950s' and qualified as a doctor in 1957 at the age of thirty-nine.[25]

During her seven years of clinical care and research on the control of pain in terminal cancer at St Joseph's Hospice, in the impoverished East London district of Hackney, Saunders found that 70 per cent of patients referred from hospitals or from their homes, at the point when active treatment was deemed no longer necessary, were in advanced stages of late-diagnosed cancer and had been suffering prolonged periods of pain severe enough to be in need of narcotics. Observing that pain relief at St Joseph's was administered on demand rather than regularly, Saunders established a clinical routine of regular analgesia and recording. Chillingly, Saunders's example of insisting on access to medication as the first step in alleviating the unnecessary suffering of her patients would inspire the Sackler family to produce their first painkiller, initially without the approval of the US Food and Drug Administration, a morphine pill named MS Contin, launched in the 1970s. (The drug went on to generate $70 million dollars a year in sales.)[26] The staggering irony here is that, for Saunders, the very 'use of the word pain', as she explains in 'The Philosophy of Terminal Care', in all her lifetime's work was 'a deliberate attempt to stimulate students and others to look at the various facets of a dying patient's distress, beyond the requirement for analgesics, to the need for human understanding and practical human help'.[27] Thus, in addition to routinized medication, Saunders innovated a research methodology 'of simple listening, recording and analysing',[28] including the keeping of a pain diary to 'give insight into what pain meant for the person [that] could be further explored by listening and talking'.[29] 'The basic methodology of listening and tape-recording, coupled with a commitment to the day-to-day care of patients with advanced malignant disease in the 45 beds, was the basis of the analysis of 1100 cases in a punch-card system (this being the pre-computer age).'[30] Saunders's unassuming description of the painstaking documentation of her encounters, which became the store of all her later work, belies the radicalism of an approach that was to prove transformational not only at St Joseph's but in the history of end-of-life care. In 1964, Saunders described an encounter that was to become definitively representative:

One person gave me more or less the following answer when I asked her a question about her pain, and in her answer she brings out the four main needs that we are trying to care for in this situation. She said, 'Well doctor, the pain began in my back, but now it seems that all of me is wrong'. She gave a description of various symptoms and ills and then went on to say, 'My husband and son were marvellous but they were at work and they would have had to stay home and lose their money. I could have cried for the pills and injections although I knew I shouldn't. Everything seemed to be against me and nobody seemed to understand'. And then she paused before she said, 'But it's so wonderful to begin to feel safe again'. Without any further questioning she had talked of her mental as well as physical distress, of her social problems and of her spiritual need for security.[31]

This kind of 'total pain', wrote Saunders, 'has physical, mental, social and spiritual elements'. 'Pain can blot out the world, cut off all true communication and perpetually renew a vicious circle of pain, fear, tension and further pain. . . . It traps the patient in a situation for which there is no reassuring explanation and to which there is no foreseeable end.'[32] For Saunders, it is the apparent unendingness of pain in (paradoxically) terminal illness that is a crucial aspect of its totalizing hold when 'when all curative and palliative measures have been exhausted':[33]

> Chronic pain of this type is not merely an extension in time of something that is essentially the same as acute pain. There is a qualitative difference. Such pain is a situation rather than an event and the hardest aspect of this situation for the patient is that it seems to be meaningless as well as endless.

For this reason, 'pain demands the same analysis and consideration as an illness itself. It is the syndromes of pain rather than the syndromes of disease with which we are concerned'.[34]

As Clark points out, '"total pain" furnished the modern hospice movement with one of its most powerful concepts'.[35] Equally influential in palliative care has been the message of Saunders's practice, and of her abundant writings, lectures and interviews, that 'total pain' demands total *care*: 'Neither she in her words nor we in our approach and treatment can deal with any of these separately.'[36] When, following almost a decade of fundraising, Saunders established, in 1967, St Christopher's, the first hospice to be founded on these ground-breaking principles, years of experience had taught her that both clinically and methodologically the emphasis must be 'multiprofessional'[37] and multi-dimensional. Nonetheless, though 'palliative care may begin with symptom control . . . in most cases that is only the beginning'.[38] 'The spiritual needs of patients and families struggling with what might seem pointless suffering were a greater challenge. Fear and grief were often inarticulate.'[39]

> Above all, no one should let himself be tempted into believing that because the patient's expectation of dying is not expressed, it is not in his mind. If it is already there he may be seeking to unburden himself and will not suffer embarrassment. Surely the doctor whom he trusts should not be the one to deny him the unhurried opportunity.[40]

Saunders asserted that 'the automatic prescribing of antidepressant drugs or tranquillizers is to be deprecated; grief is appropriate and the understanding of suffering and its creative handling may be as important as attempts at its alleviation'.[41] 'If you listen to the tale of each one and treat it separately, you will have so much less need for sedatives, tranquillisers and even analgesics.'[42] As Clark points out, 'This is a medicine concerned also for the meaning of pain' (quoting Saunders): 'A cry just to be rid of pain is not worthy of man. . . . Man by his very nature finds that he has to question the pain he endures and seek meaning in it.'[43]

Religious conviction, together with a tradition of religious charity, helped found the modern hospice movement and the recognition of palliative care as a clinical specialism. This origin confounds to some degree the historical picture of pain care and alleviation as being increasingly annexed to medicine as opposed to religion. But more broadly, this narrative attests, as I suggested above, to the widely recognized failure of modern medical approaches to take account of the demand for meaning in non-reductive ways.[44] It is striking, in this regard, how closely, and almost exactly contemporaneously, Saunders's problems and solutions to pain echo those of Michael Balint, whose 'listening' practices in the context of general practice, and the generalized despair which went under the name of 'illness', helped to found the modern tradition of narrative medicine,[45] which we will encounter in Part II.

Camp pain

The second (at once practical and theoretical) model of pain and meaning, which I wish to consider in the context of what we might call the religion and secularization of pain, is that of the anthropologist Jean Jackson, author of *Camp Pain: Talking with Chronic Pain Patients*.

Jackson's work for her original and singular book (published in 2001) began in 1986, two decades after Saunders founded St Christopher's. However, in a rather neat chronology (entirely unrecognized and unintended when I first chose these two figures as representative of particular and practice-oriented stances in relation to the meaning of pain), the concept of a multidisciplinary clinic dedicated to treating chronic pain (the setting of Jackson's anthropological study and book) itself originated in the 1960s as 'the product of a growing consensus that conventional treatments for acute pain – immobilisation, opiates and heavy tranquilisers, surgical and other procedures – were often ineffective for many pain sufferers'.[46] The fact that recognition of 'total pain' existed sixty years ago in the United States, concurrently with Saunders's pioneering work in England, makes today's opioid crisis all the more alarming and incredible.

Jackson's study focused on the Commonwealth Pain Centre (CPC), which, though housed in a hospital setting, offered 'multi-disciplinary treatment . . . with emphasis on conservative non-invasive therapies'. CPC defined itself and operated as a 'therapeutic community' in which those taking part were 'active agents of therapy', not 'passive recipients of professional and bureaucratised medical care' and where patients' problems were regarded not as 'abstracted biological malfunctions but part and parcel of patients' everyday understandings and behaviour'. CPC, Jackson summarizes, 'stressed healing, not cure . . . and motivation towards healing needed to come from within'. At the core of the healing process were 'profound changes in the meaning pain had for patients at the end of their month-long stay'.[47]

Jackson occupied a unique position in relation to understanding this complex and highly individual healing process. ('Unlike the situation with chronic conditions like diabetes or alcoholism, the path of chronic pain management was not clearly marked on any map, and very different paths could and did turn out to be appropriate for different people.'[48]) First, Jackson approaches her subjects using an intense ethnographic methodology, which quickly discards the search for any tidy match between patients' responses (positive or otherwise) to the CPC programme and their overall wellbeing.

> During the fieldwork it became clear that to demonstrate correlations convincingly . . . would require filtering out much of what I was learning, because it involved puzzles, ambiguities, and misunderstandings. I came to feel that a real understanding of what CPC patients were going through would emerge more forcefully if I paid attention to these ambiguities, contradictions, and unknowns.

As Jackson recognizes, these more intractable or indefinable aspects of pain experience are not documented in clinical reports, and 'by ignoring them conventional medical and psychiatric discourses dealing with chronic pain can omit a great deal'.[49] This is my rationale for quoting extensively from Jackson's work in what follows. It is one of the few studies to have taken place in a clinical context where the subjects, in all their complex interest, have centre stage. I have only not included case studies up to this point because the psychological literature on this subject routinely omits them.

Jackson's perspective is distinctive for the further reason that she was herself a former patient of CPC. The account Jackson gives of this experience and the impact on her study is minimal and reproduced here almost in its entirety: 'For a period of three months I had severe low back pain and depression, both of which disappeared in the months following a stay at CPC. (I was seen as such a success story that the staff invited me to return and speak to a subsequent patient community.)'[50] Unable to put 'previous experiences with pain into a kind of mental deep freeze', Jackson reflexively engaged with 'the problem of sense and nonsense at the heart of the experience of severe chronic pain and pain treatment': 'My experience gave me first-hand insight, as a sensibility, a way of being in the world that seemed to require, at times, that I pay near-total attention to my bones, muscles and the like. This experiential grounding led me to ponder the cultural patterning and praxis I was realising from within my own body, including the accompanying moral implications.' As Jackson puts it, she seeks explanation 'in the sense of discovering how and why meanings were created'.[51]

Neither success in this enterprise nor a clear-cut explanation of how it happened was guaranteed. The programme's somewhat incoherent mix of 'love and acceptance' on the one hand ('people leave here knowing they are worth something and that they can do something for themselves and make life better', as one staff member put it), and of 'reality confrontation' on the other (giving verbal feedback sessions to patients about how their behaviours appear to others), produced anger, resistance and sometimes early discharge of patients. 'Even many of those who improved or saw impressive improvement in others were not sure why the treatment worked.' Patients and staff alike were agreed, however, that a key element of the programme's 'working' (when it worked) was its education of the inner life. 'It's very important', said one staff member, 'to get in touch with oneself, with how to be true to oneself and one's needs. . . . In a way [patients] are trying to give more of themselves, give themselves away to other people when they haven't given enough to themselves'. In view of the fact that those in the caring professions were 'over-represented' at CPC, the corroborating words of one patient (herself a nurse) on the critical aspect of the CPC programme are especially resonant: '[The programme involves teaching about the] whole vicious cycle . . . pain, depression, anxiety . . . narcotics . . . teaching them how to take care of themselves in an emotional way.' '"Teaching" very often meant involving patients in digging deep into their psyches, uncovering wounds that had not healed.'[52]

Jackson cites the case of Rebecca, an African-American woman in her late forties. An assistant bank manager, as well as a mother, foster-mother and grandmother, Rebecca was admitted with numbness on her left side (neck, arm and hand) which had begun with a car accident two years earlier. In the intervening period, Rebecca had undergone multiple diagnostic tests and treatments (including medication and physical therapy, such as ultrasound and massage) and an unsuccessful surgery (followed by post-operative infection). When physicians in a range of specialisms were unable to explain her condition, Rebecca had a traumatic stay in a psychiatric ward, followed by several months of serious depression. She arrived at CPC out of sheer frustration and as a last resort, highly sceptical of the psychological component of the programme. However, when a doctor referred (for a second time) to her anxiety, Rebecca had a sudden 'breakthrough'. (Jackson quotes Rebecca as follows):

Something in the back of my mind was, like – it was more of a challenge than anything, because I thought '[the doctor's] trying to tell you something deeper than the way you would like it to be'. So I started thinking about it and it hit me right in the back of my head like a cast iron skillet: 'you know what it is, you know what it is!'

Jackson explains that '[Rebecca] did not tell me what "it" was, nor did I ask, although it seemed likely, as we talked, that she was referring to some kind of childhood abuse, probably sexual, by a man'. Quoting Rebecca again –

That one thing was a problem that, subconsciously, I simply did not acknowledge . . . oh gosh, for unpleasant reasons – I really didn't want to face up to it . . . never thought of it in the context of it having anything to do with my pain: it was totally disassociated from that in my way of thinking. . . . Acknowledging it also means that I am going to have to really work at it: just saying it is not enough. I'm going to have to dig kind of deep inside myself to get rid of it, and the problem is hostility and anger and the feeling of having been abandoned. So it's something I have to work at but the hardest part is done . . . admitting it to myself.[53]

There were two consequences of Rebecca's acknowledgement of what had previously been inadmissible. Firstly, although Rebecca 'knew she was not going to get rid of the pain', there was, nonetheless, 'a way for her to get rid of the anger, the hostility and the feeling of abandonment, which would give her a greater chance of being able to cope with the pain'. Secondly, and relatedly, she was able to describe her pain: 'Since the accident, I always felt there was a tall, dark figure behind me, always. I could look over and it was there, kind of looming.' Realizing that the figure represented 'the pain and my fear of it', Rebecca recounted how she had 'taken the cloak away and invited him to stop hanging over my shoulder and have a seat right here beside me'. At the point of leaving CPC, Rebecca reported that 'her level of pain had not changed but her ability to recognise and accept it and live in spite of it had greatly changed'.

Rebecca said her pain was like a heavy weight, an anvil, and that after her flash of insight she had a sense of 'taking the anvil and not even lifting up, but, it's like when you sit for a long time . . . you still can't get up and walk around, but you can kind of shift the weight and it gives you a little bit of comfort'. The anvil was still there, but 'getting it off of one shoulder will do me good'.[54]

Jackson describes Rebecca (significantly in the context of the emphasis of this section of the present book) as a 'CPC convert', self-consciously using the analogy of religious conversion as a conceptual tool for understanding the shift in interpretation: 'because for some patients the CPC experience cannot be explained in terms of learning new information during workshops, classes and informal conversations, or in terms of the effect of psychotherapy'. Though sceptical as to whether CPC converts underwent the fundamental shift in their 'sense of ultimate grounding' or 'root reality' conventionally associated with religious converts, the radical personal change which characterized CPC transformations in their relation to their pain, says Jackson, resembled aspects of faith conversion. 'Biographical reconstruction', for example, occurred 'in the sense that, prior to admission, pain had dominated their lives, but on discharge they had a new explanation for their pain and accompanying problems . . . reported a decreased level of suffering (some, not all, reported a decreased level of pain), and testified to a fundamental change in the degree to which pain dominated their lives'. In addition, 'a major shift in thinking about the causes of pain is characteristic', including 'acceptance of internal factors, . . . and, concomitantly, [that] one was responsible for how one experienced the pain to some degree'. Thus, while, a patient such as Rebecca (like all CPC residents) came to the programme seeking to be free of pain, at least one staff member 'was not sure to what degree that happened or to what degree that was even important. . . . Pain doesn't have to be suffering – the sensory output and how it's perceived and interpreted and how it gets translated to pain' was what mattered. Jackson goes further to hypothesize that "'seekers' are more likely to undergo conversion precisely because they are in active pursuit of just such self-transformation":

> CPC converts were on a quest for a kind of meaning that was absent in a very significant part of their lives, an absence that troubled them greatly. . . . To some extent, then, CPC converts did undergo a change in values, beliefs, and identity features significant enough to change some features of the universe of discourse – to become in some ways 'true believers'.[55]

William James's account of conversion in *The Varieties of Religious Experience* is instructive here, since, like Jackson's, it takes individual human case studies for its raw 'data' and likewise rests on the fault line between belief and psychology. James writes of Saint Augustine's aspirations to a purer life as representing 'the simultaneous coexistence of two or more different groups of aims, of which one practically holds the right of way and instigates activity, whilst the other's are only pious wishes, and never practically come to anything'. The pious wishes 'exist on the remoter outskirts of the mind, and the real self of the man, the centre of his energies, is occupied with an entirely different system'. In undergoing his conversion, Augustine's centre 'stands now planted in what was once for it a practically unreal object, and speaks from it as from its proper habitat and centre'. Such 'transformation' is only a more dramatic example of 'our ordinary alterations of character as we pass from one of our aims to another'.

> There is a constant change of our interests, and a consequent change of place in our systems of ideas, from more central to more peripheral, and from more peripheral to more central parts of consciousness. . . . [In each change there is found a part] which figures as focal and contains the excitement, and from which, as from a centre, the aim seems to be taken. Talking of this part, we involuntarily apply words of perspective to distinguish it from the rest, words like 'here', 'this', 'now', 'mine', or 'me'; and we ascribe to the other parts the positions 'there', 'then', 'that', 'his' or 'thine', 'it', 'not me'. But a 'here' can change to a 'there', and a 'there' become a 'here', and what was 'mine' and what was 'not mine' change their places. What brings such changes about is the way in which emotional excitement alters. Things hot and vital to us to-day are cold to-morrow.

The 'hot' parts are the centres of our dynamic energy, 'whereas the cold parts leave us indifferent and passive in proportion to their coldness'. To say that a person is 'converted', then, means that ideas previously peripheral to consciousness now become *the habitual centre of [one's] personal energy*.[56] James's account of the process mirrors almost exactly the report of patients and carers at CPC – that the happening was as sudden and conventionally inexplicable as it was involuntarily a shift from 'not me' to 'me' ('It hit me right in the back of the head', as Rebecca put it), a 'there' become a 'here', and 'now':

> Neither an outside observer nor the Subject who undergoes the process can explain fully how particular experiences are able to change one's centre of energy so decisively, or why they so often have to bide their hour to do so. We have a thought, or we perform an act, repeatedly, but on a certain day the real meaning of the thought peals through us for the first time, or the act has suddenly turned into a moral impossibility. All we know is that there are dead feelings, dead ideas, and cold beliefs, and there are hot and live ones; and when one grows hot and alive within us, everything has to re-crystallize about it.[57]

The analogy, or rather affinity, between Jackson's and James's accounts of conversion in religion and in psychology holds because in religious seekers, as in those seeking relief from pain at CPC, there is both a 'conscious and voluntary way and an involuntary and unconscious way in which mental results get accomplished':

> Conscious wit and will, so far as they strain towards the ideal, are aiming at something only dimly and inaccurately imagined. Yet all the while the forces of mere organic ripening within are going on towards their own prefigured result, and conscious strainings are letting loose subconscious allies behind the scenes, which in their way work towards rearrangement.[58]

This shift in the organizing centre of energies happening beneath but also in accordance with the conscious will to change perhaps helps to explain not only the converts to CPC in Jackson's study, but the success, as we saw in Chapter 1, of CBT, or prayer, in some rather than others. It is an explanation that rests on what James called, writing in 1902, 'the most important step forward' since he became a student of psychology and the evolution of which founded the CPC programme of psychological treatment: the discovery of 'whole systems of underground life . . . buried outside of the primary fields of consciousness, and making irruptions thereinto with hallucinations, pains, convulsions, paralyses of feeling and of motion, and the whole procession of symptoms of . . . disease of body and of mind'.[59] It is to this revolution, and the influence of psychoanalysis in the understanding and approach to physical symptoms of pain, that I now turn.

3

Pain: Body and mind

Jackson concludes of the CPC programme, 'In sum, the milieu itself did not necessarily produce improvement':

> Rather, its power to pitch patients more deeply into the ambiguities led them to affirm the pain paradox, which is that one's pain is absolutely real but must be treated as in the mind. This is what really made the difference, and it had to happen this way because of our Cartesian legacy of radical mind/body separation.[1]

The emphasis in Jackson's work, as in Saunders's ('all of me is wrong'), on the *in*separability of mind and body is wholly in keeping with thinking around pain from almost every discipline. The difference with Jackson's and Saunders's thinking is that the mind/body issue is encountered not as a thorny theoretical matter only, but as a defining aspect of specific human instances of the struggle with pain. 'CPC worked (*when* it worked) because patients confronted and dealt with the pain paradox on an individual basis.'[2] CPC relies, as we have seen, on a psychodynamic legacy dating back to Freudian psychoanalysis, arguably the area of enquiry where mind/body dualism in relation to individual experience (rather than as a philosophical paradox) has been most painstakingly addressed. To give an example.

A 24-year-old woman whom I will call Liz has been experiencing extreme pain while walking for over two years and is quickly overwhelmed by tiredness even when standing. The pain is most intense in one thigh, though it spreads to the whole of both legs intermittently. Since medical examination shows the reflex and range of movement of the limbs to be sound, there is no organic explanation for the pain, which began in the months before her father's death from heart disease. Liz, who had been very close to her father, had become his primary carer during his final illness and the demands of the role had prevented her from continuing a relationship with a young man to whom she was warmly attached and had hopes of a future. Liz's doctor concludes that there is a strong probability the pain originated from common muscular rheumatic pains caused by nursing her father around the clock during a cold winter when she was frequently woken by his calls in the middle of the night, and when her diet, exercise and sleep patterns were poor. The right thigh from which the pain issued was the place where her father rested his badly swollen leg so that Liz could change the bandage every day. Although, over the following two years – during which Liz cared for her unwell mother – the pain ceased, it reappeared when she was recuperating from the exhaustion of this period of care by taking a holiday with her mother and two recently married elder sisters and their husbands. When one of her much-loved sisters fell ill and died from congenital heart disease aggravated by pregnancy, Liz was again her carer, and, during this emotionally charged time, conceived tender feelings for her brother-in-law. For the past eighteen months, with her loved ones either dead or living at a distance, Liz, the pain in her legs now constantly severe, has been secluded in grief with her mother.[3]

It will be obvious to many readers by now that this is a thinly disguised summary of Freud's famous case study of Fraulein Elisabeth von R, the patient who was the occasion of Freud's 'first full-length analysis of a hysteria'[4] and thus of the founding of psychoanalytic theory and practice. I have begun by drawing the bare, spare outlines of this case, firstly, to show how, as Freud himself puts it, this 'tale of suffering' with which 'we cannot refrain from deep human sympathy' is, from a medical or curative point of view, 'made up of commonplace emotional upheavals': 'There was nothing about it to explain why it was particularly from hysteria that she fell ill . . . or why her hysteria took [this] particular form.'[5] The whole tradition of psychoanalysis, it seems, grew out of a question and problem faced by Freud as a physician over a century ago, which confronts medical practitioners on a daily basis in the modern world. I present the case in this way, secondly, therefore, in order to rehearse Freud's conclusions about the causes of Fraulein Elisabeth von R's pain as if this were indeed a 'commonplace' case: not, that is, the foundation of a theory that changed the Western world's understanding of the psyche forever; but what it undisputedly remains – the intimate and individualized understanding of personal suffering, which could be that of a contemporary person living with chronic pain in a twenty-first century version of CPC.

Below is a potted summary of Freud's conclusions, using exclusively Freud's own words:

> While the patient was nursing her father, the circle of ideas embracing her duties to her sick parent came into conflict with the content of erotic desire

she was feeling at the time. Under the pressure of lively self-reproaches, she decided in favour of the former, the erotic idea was repressed from association and the affect attaching to that idea was used to intensify or revive a physical pain which was present simultaneously or shortly before. What happened then was the prototype of the later events which led to the outbreak of her illness. The patient had formed an association between her painful mental impressions and the bodily pains which she happened to be experiencing at the time, and now, in her life of memories, she was using her physical feelings as a symbol for her mental ones. Her motives for making a substitution of this kind was the repudiation of her erotic thoughts towards her brother in law whose acceptance into her consciousness was resisted by her whole moral being. She succeeded in sparing herself the painful conviction that she loved her sister's husband by inducing physical pains in herself instead.[6]

Here, Freud describes the classic model of 'hysterical conversion': 'the "fending" off of an incompatible idea through the conversion of psychical excitations into something physical'.

We may ask: what is it that turns into physical pain here? A cautious reply would be: something that might have become, and should have become, mental pain. . . . The motive was that of defence, the refusal on the part of the patient's whole ego to come to terms with this ideational group. The mechanism was that of conversion: i.e. in place of the mental pains which she avoided, physical pains made their appearance. In this way a transformation was effected which had the advantage that the patient escaped from an intolerable mental condition; though, it is true, this was at the cost of a psychical abnormality – the splitting of consciousness that came about – and of a physical illness – her pains.[7]

An unwanted thought is 'split off' from consciousness and 'converted' into a physical symptom. The translation to physical pain spares the individual from a more unbearable mental one – the entry into consciousness of an inadmissible idea – and is thereby driven underground, wilfully forgotten, inhibited, suppressed rather than 'abreacted'[8] (expressed and consequently released). As the subject of another of Freud's famous case studies (Lucy R) put it: '"I didn't know – or rather I didn't want to know. I wanted to drive it out of my head and not think of it again."' 'I have never managed to give a better description than this', Freud wrote, 'of the strange state of mind in which one knows and does not know a thing at the same time'.[9]

A further compelling aspect of Fraulein Elisabeth's case history, in view of the previous chapter, is that she was (albeit as a family member) a sick-nurse, a role which 'for good reason', Freud and Breuer conclude, 'plays . . . a significant part in the prehistory of cases of hysteria'. Aside from the 'obvious' factors (neglect of one's own health, disturbed sleep, 'constant worry'), 'the most important determinant is to be looked for elsewhere':

> Anyone whose mind is taken up by the hundred and one tasks of sick-nursing which follow one another in endless succession over a period of weeks and months will, on the one hand, adopt a habit of suppressing every sign of their own emotion, and on the other, will soon divert his attention away from their own impressions, since they have neither time nor strength to do justice to them. Thus they will accumulate a mass of impressions which are capable of affect, which are hardly sufficiently perceived and which, in any case, have not been weakened by abreaction. [When] the period of mourning sets in, during which the only things that seem to have value are those that relate to the person who has died, these impressions that have not yet been dealt with come into the picture as well; and after a short interval of exhaustion the hysteria, whose seeds were sown during the time of nursing, breaks out.[10]

The endurance of caring creates 'material for a retention hysteria', 'an abreaction of arrears'.[11] The connection with Jackson's finding that carers are over-represented in the chronic pain community is resonant indeed. The pain is a debt to unresolved, unexpressed and unacknowledged emotional suffering. The conclusion can be extrapolated, of course, to the many forms of subjection to distress and suffering which, as we saw in Chapter 1, arguably account for chronic pain.

The identification of the hysterical symptom as the substitute formation for erotic content, and thus as the founding cornerstone of Freudian theory, has tended to obscure key insights of *Studies in Hysteria* in relation to the possible reasons for the *chronicity* of chronic pain – its ongoingness. For one thing, not knowing, avoiding, escaping, making bearable, is not the accomplishment of one occasion of conversion only but a labour requiring constant vigilance, because 'consciousness, plainly, does not know in advance when an incompatible idea is going to crop up'. Indeed, 'the incompatible idea . . . must originally have been in communication with the main stream of thought. Otherwise the conflict which led to their exclusion could not have taken place':

> An experience similar to the one which originally introduced the incompatible idea adds fresh excitation to the separated psychical group and so puts a temporary stop to the success of the conversion. The ego is obliged to attend to this sudden flare-up of the idea and to restore the former state of affairs by a further conversion.[12]

(I note in passing that 'flare-up' is the common term among chronic pain sufferers and those who treat them for intermittent intensities of pain.) In the case of Fraulein Elisabeth, being much in the company of her brother-in-law made her 'particularly liable to the occurrence of fresh traumas':

> In this way, firstly, the painful region had been extended by the addition of adjacent areas: every fresh theme which had a pathogenic effect had cathected a new region in the legs; secondly, each of the scenes which made a powerful impression on her had left a trace behind it, bringing about lasting and constantly accumulating cathexis of the various functions of the legs, a linking of these functions with her feelings of pain.[13]

'Constantly accumulating'. While the cure consists of 'one affective recollection' (under hypnosis or in therapy), the suffering itself is from 'reminiscen*ces*' (plural). The pains produced by the conversion ensued not from the 'impressions when they were fresh' of her first period of sick-nursing but from subsequent 'memories' of those same impressions.[14] 'Almost invariably when I have investigated the determinants of such conditions', says Freud, 'what I have come upon has not been a *single* traumatic cause but a group of similar ones'. This 'incontrovertible fact of the summation of traumas' means that conversion can equally 'proceed on the strength of recollected affects as well as fresh ones'. Moreover, this 'postulate' of conversion 'does no more than bring the behaviour of hysterical people nearer to that of healthy ones':

> There is no doubt that the continued existence in consciousness of ideas whose affect has not been dealt with can be tolerated by healthy individuals up to a great amount. What we are concerned with is clearly a quantitative factor – the question of how much affective tension of this kind an organism can tolerate. Even a hysteric can retain a certain amount of affect that has not been dealt with; if, owing to the occurrence of similar provoking causes, that amount is increased by summation to a point beyond the subject's tolerance, the impetus to conversion is given.[15]

There is more than a semantic link here between the 'summation of traumas' ('constantly accumulating') and the cumulative load we encountered in Chapter 1. Freud's conclusion that 'a quantitative factor' – the 'amount' of trauma relative to individual tolerance of it – is all important in marking the distinction between health and chronic illness is wholly consonant with the recognized range of determinants in current understandings of chronic pain. I press the point because of the strong pertinence, in addition, of a further 'mechanism' which Freud identifies in Fraulein Elisabeth's case as 'unmistakably involved in the building up of his patient's inability to stand and walk'. The patient's story concluded with her complaint that the episodes she had described, including unsuccessful attempts to establish a new life for her family, 'had made the fact of her standing alone painful to her':

> She was never tired of repeating that what was painful about them had been her feeling of helplessness, the feeling that she could not take a single step forward. . . . The patient [had found] . . . a somatic expression for her lack of an independent position and her inability to make any alteration in her circumstances. . . . Such phrases as 'not being able to take a single step forward', 'not having anything to lean upon', served as the bridge for this fresh act of conversion. [The condition] which was already present received considerable reinforcement in this way.[16]

This is a version of the psychic-physical feedback loops we encountered in Chapter 1, with helplessness and pain recreating one another. In *Why Psychoanalysis?*, Elisabeth Roudinesco writes: 'Of course hysteria has not disappeared, but it is increasingly experienced and treated as a form of depression – the psychical epidemic of democratic societies.'[17] It might be argued that the epidemic of chronic pain, too, like its close relation, depression, 'is the late twentieth century equivalent of hysteria'.[18] Indeed, according to Freud's theory, chronic pain is the *more likely* expression of helplessness as it has something 'to go on' as it were. In seeking to explain why Fraulein Elisabeth's mental pain came to be represented by pains in the legs rather than elsewhere, he said:

> The circumstances indicate that somatic pain was not created by the neurosis but merely *used, increased and maintained* by it. I may add at once that I have found a similar state of things in almost all the instances of hysterical pains into which I have been able to obtain an insight. There had always been a genuine, organically-founded pain present at the start. It is the commonest and most widespread human pains that seem to be most often chosen to play a part in hysteria.[19]

* * *

The most significant and influential twentieth-century afterlife of *Studies* in relation to pain was George Engel's landmark essay, published in 1959, in which he defined 'psychogenic' pain. 'What is experienced and reported as pain is a psychological phenomenon. Pain does not come into being without the operation of the psychic mechanisms which give rise to its identifiable qualities and which permit its perception. In neurophysiological terms this also means there is no pain without the participation of higher nervous centers.'[20] The definition was based on Engel's fifteen years' experience of treating patients with diagnosed and undiagnosed pain disorders as a researcher and attending physician on wards at university medical centres in the United States. The trace of *Studies* is strong in Engel's accounts of, for example: the unconscious revival of a past pain experience (an injury, operation or physical disorder) whereby the patient 'by mechanisms not understood suffers again from pain of the same character and in the same location as the original pain . . . which had occurred at a time when the pain could fulfil directly or indirectly, a psychic regulating role for the patient'; and the development of pain 'following the death or any permanent loss of a loved one' where there is a 'strong element of guilt, most often related to ambivalence toward the lost person'.

> Once the psychic organization necessary for pain has evolved, the experience, pain, no longer requires peripheral stimulation to be provoked, just as visual and auditory sensations (hallucinations) may occur without sense organ input. When such are projected outside the mind (in contrast to a painful thought or a painful frame of mind) they are felt as being in some part of the body and are to the patient indistinguishable from pain arising in the periphery.[21]

While 'the largest percentage' of the incidences Engel encounters 'follow the classic model of the hysterical conversion mechanism, in which the pain simultaneously expresses symbolically the forbidden impulse and at the same time prevents it being acted upon',[22] Engel's definition is also heavily inflected by twentieth-century (largely British) evolutions of Freud's psychic models: in particular, object relations theory and the emphasis of Melanie Klein and Donald W. Winnicott on the role of interpersonal relationships – especially parent-child attachment – and their unconscious internalizations in infant development and psychic organization. For example, among Engel's several vignettes of the experience of face pain is one in which an adult daughter is afflicted by her mother's deathbed pain when she is finally free to marry her fiancé. 'Sometimes the site of the pain is determined by a conscious or unconscious wish that the other person suffer pain . . . the patient inflicting on herself exactly what she wished on the other person.'[23] These determinants of pain location are to be understood, says Engel, in terms of the importance of interpersonal relations in preserving 'psychic balance': 'They are expressions par excellence of attempts to maintain object relations, albeit at a price.'[24] A predisposition towards these developments was associated with 'distressing experiences' in childhood, 'where aggression, suffering and pain played an important role in early family relationships'. In cases of actual or threatened loss of the object, 'It is as if the patient says, "If I can't continue to have this relationship and get from it what I want and need, I will become like them in some way" thus experiencing the object's pain, real or fantasied'.[25] As we have seen, Engel's observation of the strong association between chronic pain and a history of childhood trauma and abuse has been vindicated by a wealth of research in more recent decades.

Engel is fulsome in acknowledging the debt his theory and practice owe to *Studies in Hysteria* and urges his profession to follow his lead in reading the 'richly rewarding . . . wealth of case material' to learn at first-hand 'the nature of the data and observations which permitted Freud to discover how pain may develop as a purely psychic phenomenon'. Engel asserts that 'every physician is free to rediscover for themselves what Freud discovered about pain if they follow two simple principles: permit the patients to talk freely and take seriously what the patient says', as much about their lives, families and relationships as about themselves. The key is not to 'force a separation between what is regarded as organic and what is regarded as psychological or social':

> This is more economical in time and expense for both the physician and the patient than the currently traditional technic of 'ruling out organic disease' and attempting to establish a diagnosis by exclusion. Such interminable diagnostic procedures may not only be a waste of time and money but may also render virtually impossible the establishment of correct diagnosis simply because the patient themselves becomes increasingly oriented towards this type of approach and less spontaneous in revealing personal and psychological data which the physician, by their approach and behaviour, has made them feel are completely out of place.

Engel makes this plea as part of a concluding 'historical note' in which he confesses himself astounded that Freud's case studies' contribution to the understanding of pain has had 'so little influence on medicine in general' such that 'the analyst or psychiatrist is rarely consulted directly by a patient because of pain and only infrequently are such patients referred'. From the vantage point of the 1950s, Engel explains this state of affairs by the reluctance of both physicians and patients to view their pain as psychological. 'Pain patients in particular are among the most reluctant to accept a psychiatric referral and to participate in psychotherapy if they do so. In general, they regard their symptoms as organic in origin, a belief in which they are often supported by their physicians.'[26]

Skip forward almost sixty years to the situation described by a psychiatrist at the opening of a paper for the *Journal of the American Academy of Psychoanalysis and Dynamic Psychiatry* in 2008:

Although patients with medically unexplained chronic pain are sometimes referred for psychiatric consultation, it is rare for them to be recommended for a psychoanalytically informed treatment. . . . The paucity of referrals to psychoanalysts may be attributed partly to a mind–body split in which chronic pain is defined by most physicians, patients, and our culture as primarily a biomedical condition. It may also reflect a lack of interest among psychoanalysts in treating such cases. Patients with chronic pain syndromes [because they experience their pains as primarily physical] can be difficult to engage in the analytic process and require much patience and flexibility on the part of the analyst.[27]

Patients and doctors do not want to see chronic pain as psychic, and psychoanalysts are reluctant to treat it as such. That this state of affairs continues into modern-day practice is all the more surprising for two reasons.

Firstly, while (as is frequently acknowledged), 'there is relatively little psychoanalytic literature on the subject of chronic pain',[28] psychodynamic ideas have never ceased to influence thinking about chronic pain. A substantial body of work has grown up, for example – heavily influenced by John Bowlby's attachment theory,[29] and frequently citing Engel's work (especially the strong association he found between childhood neglect or abuse and chronic pain) – around the relationship between chronic pain and attachment. Lawrence C. Kolb, while a psychiatrist at the Veterans Administration Medical Centre in New York, in 1982, asserted that persistent pain in many adults is 'one of the expressions of continuing attachment behaviour – an attempt to elicit caretaking behaviour'.[30] In 1994, Anderson and Hines claimed that 'chronic pain often represents a nonspecific plea for help in overcoming earlier unresolved trauma, traumas that have disrupted the most basic of human needs – a secure attachment'.[31] In the same year, Mikail, Henderson and Tasca proposed that the focus of psychosocial assessment and treatment 'be extended beyond the current emphasis on coping and emotional functioning to include determination of patients' attachment styles and patterns within previous and current interpersonal relationships'.[32] These theories have been corroborated, updated and formalized by recent research,[33] with a 2016 review of literature on chronic pain in children and adolescents concluding that 'Complex early interactions between a child's developing self-regulatory systems and their caregiver's responses may impact on the vulnerability, onset and offset, or maintenance of chronic pain. Given that a significant proportion of children and adolescents experiencing chronic and recurrent pains subsequently experience persistence of such into adulthood the influence of enduring attachment patterns may be particularly important'.[34] But the very reiteration of these ideas (still speculatively) as a *theoretical* framework on which to base treatment and practice suggests that the latter have changed little[35] since Perlman wrote in 1996: 'I have worked with many incest and child-abuse survivors who were treated for years for physical disorders. On analytic treatment, these physical disorders have often turned out to be, in the patient's view and mine, the body memories of physical and sexual abuse.'[36]

The second reason that the absence of psychoanalytic treatment of chronic pain appears curious is the increasing neuroscientific interest in 'the conversion of emotional problems into physical symptoms'[37] including functional imaging findings that suggest involvement of the PFC in the neural mechanisms of 'conversion disorder'[38] (the term derived from Freud's theory of mental pain turned physical). The findings are intriguingly pertinent to the association of PFC restructuring with chronic pain, which we saw in Chapter 1, and suggest that neuroscience is in some ways catching up with psychoanalytic theory. Indeed, consultant neurologist Suzanne O'Sullivan claims in her award-winning *It's All in Your Head: Stories from the Frontline of Psychosomatic Illness* that, 'for all the shortcomings in the concepts proposed by Freud and Breuer in *Studies*, the twenty-first century has brought no great advances to a better understanding of the mechanisms for this disorder'.[39] Even so, as O'Sullivan points out, in the *DSM*, the classificatory system of mental disorders published by the American Psychiatric Association, now in its fifth iteration and the 'bible' of psychological and psychiatric illness, 'the term psychosomatic disorder does not appear'.[40] Neither does the term chronic pain.

The history of the categorization of chronic pain in the *DSM* is instructive in relation to the fate of the condition vis-à-vis psychoanalysis and its treatment more generally. *DSM-3*, published in 1980, introduced a psychiatric entity for chronic pain within a newly established diagnostic spectrum of 'somatoform disorders' – which included conversion disorder – called 'psychogenic pain disorder'.[41] The concept of 'psychogenic' pain had been widely adopted during the two or three preceding decades, bolstered by Engel's classic 1959 paper discussed above. The classification was subsequently revised to 'somatoform pain disorder'[42] but both terms were dropped in *DSM-4*, published in 1994, on the basis that they reinforced an outdated Cartesian dualism which had been superseded for pain specialists by the neuromatrix model of pain, proposed by Melzack and now widely accepted, as we saw in Chapter 1. As explained there, the neuromatrix theory postulates that the experience of pain is a complex interaction of sensory, affective and cognitive components, in which the brain is actively involved, generating and modulating pain in response to, and independent of, sensory input. 'It is no longer possible to argue for discrete "organic" and "psychogenic" etiologies of pain', assert Gagliese and Katz, in their boldly titled tribute to Melzack, 'Medically Unexplained Pain is not Caused by Psychopathology'. 'Within this framework, pain that arises from thoughts and feelings is normal and not an indication of psychopathology or psychiatric illness.' Aside from their criticism of the lack of empirical evidence 'to prove that psychopathology causes pain and . . . to specify the mechanisms by which it is generated', the authors strongly object to 'the practice of relegating certain inexplicable phenomena to the psychological or emotional realm', for the reason that it is 'damaging to the patient'. 'Labels such as "psychogenic" change how the individual is viewed and treated, implicitly blame him or her for the pain, . . . and introduce an element of distrust into the relationship between patient and health professional.'[43] The danger is a real one. Jackson found that patients often interpreted being referred to a psychiatrist as an implication that, for the physician, the pain was regarded as 'unfounded' and 'not real'.[44] O'Sullivan prefers the neutral term 'functional' to describe medically unexplained symptoms, aware that terms starting with the prefix 'psycho' are 'alienating' for some patients, 'particularly those who are wholly unaware of a psychological trigger'.[45] Accordingly, 'the pejorative adjectives of "psychogenic" and "somatoform"' were replaced in the *DSM-4* by 'a new, more broadly defined diagnostic grouping for pain' called 'pain disorder',[46] emphasizing psychosocial factors and providing three subtypes: pain disorder associated with psychological factors, with a general medical condition, and with both psychological factors and a general medical condition.[47] 'Pain disorder' and these subtypes were removed in the *DSM-5*, because: 'there is a lack of evidence that such distinctions can be made with reliability and validity', especially when diagnosis is (routinely) made in primary care rather than psychiatric settings; a large body of research has demonstrated that 'psychological factors influence all forms of pain'; and 'most individuals with chronic pain attribute their pain to a combination of factors, including somatic, psychological, and environmental influences'.[48] *DSM-5* includes no pain-specific disorder; rather, pain is classified under the more general Somatic Symptom Disorder, with specific diagnosis left relatively open. 'Some individuals with chronic pain would be appropriately diagnosed as having somatic symptom disorder, with predominant pain. For others, psychological factors affecting other medical conditions or an adjustment disorder would be more appropriate.'[49] While critics of the *DSM-4* classification welcome the 'expunging' of pain disorder in *DSM-5*, they protest (in some cases the same authors in the same terms) that *DSM-5*'s somatic symptom disorder 'overpsychologizes people with chronic pain; it has low sensitivity and specificity, and it contributes to misdiagnosis, as well as unnecessary stigma'. A key danger remains of 'polluting' the therapeutic relationship between provider and patient, who is 'demoralis[ed] . . . disbelieved and alone'. 'Clinicians act as though there was only one alternative. They blame faulty thinking, which for many classically-thinking doctors is the same thing as saying that there is no cause and even no disease.'[50]

These are intricate issues which I cannot hope fully to represent. But the same paradox seems to rear itself again and again. The notion of psychogenic pain, which sought to 'add' a psychological dimension to pain, as part of Engel's move towards the biopsychosocial understanding of illness, is dislodged from the *DSM* by a neuropsychological approach to pain which regards pain as 'multi-dimensional'. To the lay scholar, the two approaches (as my introduction implicitly acknowledges) seem to share remarkable affinity and common overarching aims. The to-fro debate, now correctively emphasizing psychological suffering, now re-correctively emphasizing physical suffering – always with an eye on the needs of the patient – thus effectively reproduces the Cartesian dualism it is seeking to overcome. Partly this is a symptom of medical classifications which, as Merskey points out, 'do not reflect ultimate truths and universal consistency' but are 'approximations . . . as true as the current knowledge': 'In an ideal system of classification, the categories should be mutually exclusive and completely exhaust the data to be incorporated. . . . No classification in medicine has achieved such aims and this expectation is unreasonable.' Writing in 2000, in the wake of *DSM-4*'s publication, Merskey describes chronic pain as one of the conditions which 'now lurk under the label of somatization, somatizer, or somatoform disorder' as the 'equivalent', for pain, of conversion disorder. '*DSM-4* (like the *DSM-3* system) forbids the diagnosis of conversion disorder [which directly precedes pain disorder in *DSM-3* and *-4*] for the symptom of pain. But the more it changes the more things are the same.'[51] This self-defeating effort at discrimination is compounded by the fact that the term 'somatisation', when first introduced in the mid-twentieth century, was identified with Freud's concept of conversion[52] and remains highly contested as a concept.[53]

Since Freud's legacy appears to remain central to much debate and controversy around the current understanding and treatment of chronic pain, it is worth revisiting some Freudian basics once more. Engel stated that despite pain being 'a common and prominent manifestation' of hysterical conversions, such that 'one might be justified in saying that psychoanalysis came into being through the clarification of the mechanism of some of these mysterious pain syndromes', Freud himself was 'not primarily interested in pain'.[54] According to Pontalis, however, Freud, 'without having fully developed his ideas on the subject, never ceased to interest himself in the specific problem – in his eyes, quite puzzling – that the existence of physical and psychic pain poses'.[55] Pontalis traces in Freud's work 'the outlines of an original theory of pain . . . explicitly present at both ends of his work'. In *Project for a Scientific Psychology* (1895), pain's 'first essential characteristic . . . is the phenomenon of a breaking down of barriers', 'a breach in the protective shield', occurring when, in 'an excess of excitation' or 'excessively large quantities of energy break through the protective devices'.[56] 'All sensory excitations (even those of the highest sense organs) tend to turn into pain if the stimulus increases.'[57] In *Inhibitions, Symptoms and Anxiety* (1926), this definition, as Pontalis points out, remains unchanged. 'If the pain does not proceed from a part of the skin but from an internal organ the situation is still the same. All that has happened is that a portion of the inner periphery has taken the place of the outer periphery.'[58] When Freud attempts to explain the relation of, and distinction between, pain and anxiety, however, his remarks are avowedly 'tentative' on the grounds that 'so little is known about the psychology of processes of feeling'. Freud takes as his starting-point, 'the one situation which we believe we understand' – that of the infant when presented with a stranger instead of his or her mother. That the baby 'has anxiety there can be no doubt'. But the facial expression and the reaction of crying indicate that the baby 'is feeling pain as well'. As the infant 'cannot as yet distinguish between temporary absence and permanent loss', 'as soon as [the baby] misses their mother, they behave as if they were never going to see her again'. Pain is the reaction to this 'traumatic' missing and loss of the mother, and the associated in-the-moment longing and ungratified need of the lost object; anxiety is attributable to 'the danger which that loss entails' (ultimately loss of love).[59] The 'puzzle' is this: 'The element which is essential to pain, peripheral stimulation, is entirely absent in the child's situation of longing.' 'Yet it cannot be for nothing', Freud continues, 'that the common usage of speech should have created the notion of internal pain and treated the feeling of loss of object as equivalent to physical pain'. Freud surmises as follows: when a high degree of physical pain occurs, intense 'narcissistic' energy is concentrated on the painful place, increasing until it 'tends, as it were, to empty the ego'. 'It is well known that when internal organs are giving pain, spatial and other images of the affected part of the body arise, though that part is not represented in conscious ideation on other occasions.' Freud then speculates that the conditions produced by the intense longing concentrated on the missed or lost object (one that 'steadily mounts up because it cannot be appeased') are the same as the conditions produced by the pain which is concentrated on the injured part of the body. The object longed for 'by instinctual need' 'plays the same role as the part of the body which is [breached] by an increase of [sensory] stimulus'. That is to say, 'The continuous nature of the process and the impossibility of inhibiting it produce the same state of mental helplessness'.[60] What is striking, says Pontalis, is that it is exactly the same model ('plays the same role', 'the same state of helplessness') that Freud uses to describe physical pain and psychic pain.

> There is no metaphor here, but analogy, a direct transfer from one register to another: the same words are used, the same mechanisms invoked. The experience of pain takes place within a 'body-ego'. As if, in the case of pain, the body transformed itself in to psyche and psyche into body.[61]

Pontalis's interpretation is wholly consonant with Freud's thinking in 'The Ego and the Id' published in 1923, a few years before *Inhibitions, Symptoms and*

Anxiety. 'The ego is first and foremost a bodily ego; it is not merely a surface entity, but is itself the projection of a surface':

> A person's own body, and above all its surface, is a place from which both external and internal perceptions may spring. It is seen like any other object. . . . Pain, too, seems to play a part in the process, and the way in which we gain new knowledge of our organ during painful illnesses is perhaps a model of the way by which in general we arrive at the idea of our body.[62]

The father of psychoanalysis, responsible for situating pain in the mind, says that self, mind and ego start in the *body*, and start *with pain*! And that first pain is the most instinctual, most primal, most connected to our deepest emotional vulnerabilities and needs. Small wonder, then, that it can often be the first, as well as the most prolonged, mode of expression for, and the site of least resistance to, the distress of bearing one's own adult existence.

Moreover, in his own study of psychosomatic illness in the second half of the twentieth century, Winnicott added a further compelling dimension, of relevance to chronic pain, to Freud's explanation of how 'the ego is based on the body-ego'.

> Freud might have gone on to say that in health the self retains this seeming identity with the body and its functioning. [Out of] a functioning body there develops a functioning personality, complete with defences against anxiety of all degrees and kinds. [This] is the inherited tendency of each individual to achieve a unity of the psyche and the soma, an experiential identity of the spirit or psyche and the totality of physical functioning.

At one level, says Winnicott, 'psychosomatic illness implies a split in the individual's personality, with weakness of the linkage between psyche and soma'. Yet, at another level, 'there remains in the individual ill person . . . a tendency not altogether to lose the psycho-somatic linkage'.

> Here, then, is the positive value of somatic involvement. The individual values the potential psycho-somatic linkage which protects . . . from a flight into an intellectualized or a spiritual existence, or into compulsive [behaviours] which would ignore the claims of a psyche that is built and maintained on a basis of somatic functioning.

In this way, 'psycho-somatic illness is the negative of a positive – the tendency towards integration'.[63] This seems an aspect of chronic pain that has been overlooked. That is to say, as a symptom, it guards against more extreme forms of dissociation or disintegration, by preserving the 'healthy' inclination towards a unity of body and mind.

4

Pain and language

At the close of his case study on Fraulein Elisabeth, Freud shows an early interest in 'the common usage of speech' in relation to pain, which we encountered in his later work at the close of Chapter 3. He concludes in *Studies* that 'somatic expression depends less than one would imagine on personal or voluntary factors':

> How has it come about that we speak of someone who has been slighted as being 'stabbed to the heart' unless the slight had in fact been accompanied by a precordial sensation which could suitably be described in that phrase and unless it was identifiable by that sensation? What could be more probable than that the figure of speech 'swallowing something', which we use in talking of an insult to which no rejoinder has been made, did in fact originate from the innervatory sensations which arise in the pharynx when we refrain from speaking and prevent ourselves from reacting to the insult? . . . These may now for the most part have become so much weakened that the expression of them in words seems to us only to be a figurative picture of them, whereas in all probability the description was once meant literally.

Thus, Freud concludes, taking a verbal expression literally and feeling the 'stab in the heart' as a real event 'is not taking liberties with words, but is simply reviving once more the sensations to which the verbal expression owes its justification'.[1] Freud's compelling suggestion, spanning his interest in pain, is that the everyday, conventionalized language of pain is not merely secondary or cliched in its expression of pain, but originates in, and even 'revives', painful bodily sensation. This notion keeps alive the mind/body nexus, here at the close of Part I, as I turn to confront the issue of language and pain, as a prelude to considering the role of *literary* language in relation to *chronic* pain in Part II. In what follows, I draw, broadly speaking, on three perspectives

– philosophical, psychological and psychoanalytical – which, as will become self-evident, often wittingly overlap.

It is de rigueur for scholars of pain from multiple disciplines to take as a starting-point Elaine Scarry's central contention, in her ground-breaking work, *The Body in Pain: The Making and Unmaking of the World*, as to the radical incommunicability of pain, its central entailment of the 'shattering of language'. First 'complaint . . . becomes the exclusive mode of speech' until 'eventually the pain so deepens that the coherence of complaint is displaced by . . . reversion to a state anterior to language, to the sounds and cries a human being makes before language is learned'.[2] Think, as Scarry directs us to do, of King Lear on the heath, reduced, in Freud's terms, to pain's primal stabs and grunts, cries that precede the making and learning of language.[3] While this aspect of Scarry's compelling thesis has been the subject of much celebration, as well as contestation, in the four decades since its publication, it has been less common to encounter engaged dialogue with the mutually reinforcing characteristics of bodily pain which, for Scarry, render it thus destructive of the very capacity for speech.

One such characteristic is the subjective exclusiveness of pain. As Engel puts it:

> Pain falls into the category of private data-experience which cannot be simultaneously shared and reported by anyone other than the person experiencing it. . . . This is different from some varieties of experience, such as vision or hearing, where what impinges on the sense organs can also be experienced by other observers and hence some consensus can be achieved as to what was seen or heard.[4]

Scarry pursues what this phenomenon means, subjectively, for the sufferer, how this profound privacy itself *hurts*. 'To the individual experiencing it [pain is] overwhelmingly present, more emphatically real than any other human experience, and yet is almost invisible to anyone else, unfelt, and unknown.'

> The sentient fact of physical pain is not simply somewhat less easy to express than some second event, not simply somewhat less visible than some second event, but so nearly impossible to express, so flatly invisible, that the problem goes beyond the possibility that almost any other phenomenon occupying the same environment will distract attention from it. Indeed, even where it is virtually the only content in a given environment, it will be possible to describe that environment as though the pain were not there.

'By what perceptual process', Scarry asks in a question of fitting metaphysical amazement, 'does it come about that one human being can stand beside another human being in agonizing pain and not know it?'

Though indisputably real to the sufferer, it is, unless accompanied by visible body damage or a disease label, unreal to others. This profound ontological split is a doubling of pain's annihilating power: the lack of acknowledgment and recognition . . . becomes a second form of negation and rejection, the social equivalent of the physical aversiveness.

This is, Scarry points out, 'more radically true . . . of the severe and prolonged pain that may occur unaccompanied by any nameable disease'. This renders the distress for chronic pain sufferers of not being believed, which we encountered in Chapter 1, a critical and existential one.

A second characteristic is that, 'unlike any other state of consciousness', physical pain 'has no referential content':

If one were to move through all the emotional, perceptual, and somatic states that take an object – hatred for, seeing of, being hungry for – the list would become a very long one and, though it would alternate between states we are thankful for and those we dislike, it would be throughout its entirety a consistent affirmation of the human being's capacity to move out beyond the boundaries of his or her own body into the external, sharable world. This list and its implicit affirmation would, however, be suddenly interrupted when, moving through the human interior, one at last reached physical pain, for physical pain . . . is not of or for anything. It is precisely because it takes no object that it, more than any other phenomenon, resists objectification in language.[5]

Pontalis (albeit comparing pain to other psychic states) makes a startlingly similar point when he writes:

I *have* anxiety, I *am* pain. . . . At least anxiety can be expressed, can be coined into the formation of symptoms, can modulate itself into representations and phantasies, or discharge itself through acting out. It can even be contagious, whereas pain belongs only to oneself. Anxiety remains communicable, an indirect appeal to another; pain can only be cried out.

'This cry', Pontalis goes on, 'does nothing to assuage it – only to fall back into silence where it becomes one with the being'.[6] Or as Scarry puts it: 'Nothing sustains its image in the world; nothing alerts us to the place it has vacated' and as such pain denies the sufferer 'the power of verbal objectification, a major source of our self-extension, a vehicle through which the pain could be lifted out into the world and eliminated'.[7]

A third characteristic is the capacity of pain to blot out everything except itself.

> It is a commonplace that at the moment when a dentist's drill hits and holds an exposed nerve, a person sees stars. What is meant by 'seeing stars' is that the contents of consciousness are, during those moments, obliterated, that the name of one's child, the memory of a friend's face, are all absent. . . . In the most literal way possible, the created world of thought and feeling, all the psychological and mental content that constitutes both one's self and one's world, and that gives rise to and is in turn made possible by language, ceases to exist.

Pain does not merely destroy language by becoming 'its only subject'.[8] By obliteration of the contents of consciousness, pain annihilates not only the objects of complex thought and emotion but also the objects of the most elemental acts of perception.

> First occurring only as an appalling but limited internal fact, it eventually occupies the entire body and spills out into the realm beyond the body, takes over all that is inside and outside, makes the two obscenely indistinguishable, and systematically destroys anything like language or world extension that is alien to itself and threatening to its claims. The most immediate and concrete objects of consciousness, have been emptied of their content. The objects of consciousness from the most expansive to the most intimate, from those that exist in the space at the very limits of vision to those that exist in the space immediately outside the boundaries of the body, – all in one patient rush are swept through and annihilated [in the] horrible momentum of this world contraction.

'Terrifying for its narrowness', Scarry concludes, 'it nevertheless exhausts and displaces all else until it seems to become the single broad and omnipresent fact of existence'.[9] Again, Pontalis's thinking is highly resonant here. As an example of the breakdown of 'the reassuring division between the physical and psychic', Pontalis refers the reader to Le Clezio's short story, 'Beaumont Acquainted with his Pain', in which a toothache is first felt as 'nothing very serious . . . just a slight pain, sharp and well-defined . . . which could be dispelled by a mere feel of an aspirin on the tongue', then 'no longer confined to a definite spot on the molar . . . this half of his jaw had suddenly become larger, in the darkness, pushing away everything around it', until finally 'this was life, a mere nothing, a vague, unvarying phenomenon, so easy to reduce; and pain, this incoherent passion . . . this new, unforeseen organ growing inside and outside himself . . . a kind of triumphal I on which the whole of his body was impaled'.[10] Pain, as Scarry puts it, 'begins by being "not oneself" and ends by having eliminated all that is "not itself"'. World, self and voice are lost, or nearly lost:

It is a state that has at its centre the single, overwhelming discrepancy between an increasingly palpable body and an increasingly substanceless world . . . an annihilating negation so hugely felt throughout [one's] own body that it overflows into the spaces before [one's] eyes and in [one's] ears and mouth; yet . . . which is unfelt, unsensed by anybody else. . . . This world unmaking, this uncreating of the created world, [the obliteration of the contents of consciousness, the elimination of world ground] which is an external objectification of the psychic experience of the person in pain, becomes itself the cause of the pain.[11]

This is the 'emptiness' which Freud describes in his conception of the body-ego in helpless pain. It is an emptiness to which this chapter and book return, almost as inevitably as the ego (healthy or otherwise) itself does.

*

Scarry's thesis that the incommunicability of pain 'doubles' its suffering arguably has its clearest counterpart in psychological and psychotherapeutic thinking in the concept of alexithymia, defined by the American Psychological Association as the 'inability to express, describe, or distinguish among one's emotions',[12] and closely associated, as we shall see, with chronic pain. The term originates, significantly, in the field of psychosomatic medicine. It was coined – from Greek roots *a* (lack), *lexis* (word), *thymos* (emotion, spirit) – by US psychiatrists John Nemiah and Peter Sifneos[13] in the second half of the twentieth century to denote the difficulty they observed among psychosomatic patients 'in finding words to describe how they feel, almost as though they did not understand the word "feeling"'.[14] In many of those reporting physiological complaints, the inability to identify and describe subjective feeling was accompanied by a style of thinking oriented towards externals. 'In reality these people knew quite little about their internal states and were often incapable of effectively relating them to memories, specific situations, or recurring fantasies.'[15] Nemiah's and Sifneos's observations and investigations converged with those of the Paris School of Psychosomatics, where contemporaneously (in the 1970s), Pierre Marty and Michel M'Uzan were identifying a form of mental functioning that might create vulnerability to the emergence of somatic disease. It was marked by 'a mechanical style of thinking – *pensée operatoire* – that is factual and non-metaphoric. . . . As these states become more or less chronic, a mechanical way of living sets in – *vie opératoire*'.[16] While the theoretical bases of these twin research endeavours were distinct,[17] their empirical findings were strongly corroborative. 'Operational thinking' was the outcome of 'the lack of a rich inner life' and a consequent 'focussing [by patients] of concerns on their organic symptoms'.[18]

The emergence of alexithymia as a construct in the 1970s was also founded on a body of US-based science and clinical evidence stretching back to the 1940s. It was influenced, for example, by the (now largely superseded) theory of neuroscientist Paul MacLean, of the brain as divided into three parts – the primitive brain (survival response), visceral brain or limbic system (emotional response) and neocortex (rational thinking and language processing). MacLean speculated that the 'apparent intellectual inability [of the patient with psychosomatic illness] to verbalize his emotional feelings' might be the result of 'little direct exchange between the visceral brain and the word brain', such that emotional feelings 'instead of being relayed to the intellect' for evaluation and symbolic expression 'might be conceived as being translated into a kind of "organ language"'.[19] MacLean's work built on that of psychiatrist Jurgen Reusch, who deduced that, when symbolic self-expression is impossible, the person 'simply gets stuck with their tension', which is manifest in the persistent physical symptom.[20] The concept of alexithymia owed much, in addition, to the psychoanalytic theory of Karen Horney and contemporaries in the 1950s. In 'The Paucity of Inner Experience', Horney describes a 'pervasive haziness of all, or most, inner experiences', in which 'the entire threshold of awareness is lowered'. It is not 'identical with an alienation from the real self, but concerns the whole actual self: the awareness of pride and self-hate, triumph and defeat, hurts, illusions. Even anger, though unmistakably shown, may not be felt as such'. Yet the paucity is not 'restricted to the emotional life – feelings of pain, of joy, of hope, of disappointment, of likes or dislikes', but 'includes thinking, willing, wishing, believing, doing. In short, it means living in a fog'. Horney goes on to give a description which indicates further how this 'fog' is distinct from the mere repression of unwanted thoughts and emotions.

> The world of inner experiences is not shriveled or extinct. Dreams that the memory retains are like the rumblings of distant volcanoes or thunderstorms and reflect the depth and aliveness of inner battles, of destruction, of despair, of attempts at some solution. But this inner world is not accessible to conscious experience. . . . It is as if the person had turned his back on his inner life . . . as if he had closed an airtight or soundproof door; as if he had walled off everything. It may be a glass wall through which he still can observe what is going on without experiencing it.

The unawareness of inner experiences is 'a severe deficiency' which 'impairs not only a person's aliveness' but 'functioning in daily life'. Horney compares it to the loss of eyesight, 'a kind of inner blindness . . . jeopardizing orientation'. As a blind person must find other ways to orient themselves in their surroundings so 'the person who is numbed to his inner experiences likewise must find other ways, and does so automatically. The most important one is to shift emphasis from the inner to the outer life'.[21] The existence of alexithymia as a phenomenon was further endorsed by the work of psychoanalyst, holocaust survivor and pioneer of mass trauma studies, Henry Krystal, who found 'disturbances of affective and cognitive patterns'[22] in his long-term follow-up of those liberated from concentration camps (among whom the rate of psychosomatic diseases was as high as 30–70 per cent).[23] Krystal concluded that what were to become known as alexithymic characteristics – 'exaggerated emphasis upon the mundane details of the "things" in one's life, and a severe impairment in the capacity for wish-fulfilment fantasy' – 'interfered with the capacity for symbolization and achievement of changes'. 'These patients do not recognize their emotions since they experience them in an undifferentiated way, poorly verbalized, and because they have very poor reflective self-awareness. As a result, they tend to complain of symptoms such as pain, palpitations or insomnia, rather than being able to form complete emotions and recognize them as "feelings". As Krystal records, 'the reconciliation of these far flung observations' of the same phenomenon[24] resulted in a consolidated model of alexithymia, with an accompanying (and, in clinical practice, widely used) assessment scale.[25] Lopez distinguishes four elementary premises: '1) difficulty in identifying and describing feelings; 2) difficulty in distinguishing between feelings and bodily sensations related to emotional activation; 3) restrained and limited imaginative processes, and 4) a cognitive style oriented toward the outside'.[26]

A range of studies have found a high prevalence, and elevated levels, of alexithymia, especially difficulties in identifying feelings, among people living with a range of chronic pain conditions.[27] There is evidence that the presence of alexithymia influences the condition, and the quality of life associated with it, in direct and indirect ways. Given the close co-occurrence of depression and alexithymia[28] – which have in common withdrawn interpersonal functioning, and reduced clarity and communication about feelings – it is possible that difficulty in identifying or expressing emotions increases symptoms of depression which in turn interferes with the person's ability to deal with pain. Alternatively, alexithymia may directly influence illness behaviour. The tendency to notice and be concerned about one's body might increase sensation magnitude and prolong or heighten physiological arousal. As a result of the inability to accurately identify subjective feelings, these sensations might be experienced as aversive physical symptoms, prompting a person to report only the undifferentiated physiological aspects of emotion.[29] The influence of alexithymia on the affective dimension of pain is strong in either case and is supported by a growing number of studies showing that suppression of emotional expression is related to significantly more symptoms of depression, increased catastrophizing, pain intensity and pain-related disability.[30]

As experts in this field point out, this evidence for a strong association between alexithymia and chronic pain is hardly surprising, given that pain is a subjective, private experience with interacting sensory and affective components, involving a proneness to experience poorly differentiated negative affects. Difficulty in identifying or communicating emotion may interact at all stages of the illness course as a precipitating, perpetuating or exacerbating factor: predisposing individuals to experience pain, triggering symptoms, modulating severity, prolonging or intensifying persistent pain or being a consequence of it or a combination of these.[31] These studies' findings offer objective confirmation of a phenomenon which is strongly present in Jean Jackson's case studies of chronic pain patients. Nurse Donna, for example, noted that most patients found it difficult to 'even notice what emotions they are feeling – just naming what they feel, that's the first one. And then once you know what you are feeling, you can choose whether or not to act out of that feeling or to act out of a different motive, a different potential'.[32]

The state of current research is by no means conclusive in terms of the precise relationship between alexithymia and chronic pain, not least because alexithymia remains a loosely defined construct from whatever view it is looked at. For example, insofar as alexithymia is conceptualized not only as 'a deficit in a person's ability to employ cognitive processes to identify, differentiate, and communicate affective states' and 'global impairment in conscious recognition of emotion', but as impeding 'successful regulation of emotions, particularly negative affects',[33] it lies somewhere between two dominant psychological concepts in clinical psychology: 'emotional regulation (or dysregulation)',[34] on the one hand (a new and growing area of research in relation to chronic pain[35]), which is concerned with a person's ability to access, be aware of, monitor and modulate emotional states and expression; and the concept of 'mentalisation',[36] on the other hand, which denotes the capacity to be aware of, think about, understand and interpret mental states – one's own and others – in terms of, for example, motivation, beliefs, needs and purposes. Moreover, because alexithymia is regarded as a broad cluster of cognitive traits, it falls outside of conventional diagnostic guidelines. It is not listed in the *DSM-5* as a mental disorder and remains a construct of some debate, partly owing to its history as an observed feature of clinical practice, which observations laid the basis for the phenomenon's definition. The consequence is that, in theoretical terms, the construct provides more 'framework' than 'precise diagnostic model',[37] a status which usefully (for my purposes) situates the concept richly at the interface of psychosomatic medicine, psychoanalysis and psychology. That is to say, the establishment and use of a standard measurement tool does not preclude from the remit of alexithymia the kind of existential inarticulacy which prompted Cicely Saunders to warn against the assumption that what is 'not expressed' is therefore 'not in mind'; nor does it exclude the life-limiting consciousness which Henry Krystal found among (prematurely) ageing holocaust survivors:

> The alexithymic becomes early prey to the most devastating pre-occupation of old age: 'Who loves me?', 'Who cares if I live?' . . . They neither experience love, nor do they have the kind of empathy which would permit them to sense their object's affection for them. One has to feel love to be able to believe in its existence. Most of all, one has to feel love in order to be able to accept one's own self and one's own past.[38]

Alexithymia also embraces, according to Taylor's history of the concept, 'the less well-known contribution'[39] of the earlier psychoanalytic theory of Wilfred Bion. As I have argued extensively elsewhere that Bion's key theory of thinking provides a powerful touchstone for a model of therapeutic reading,[40] it is to this theory that I now turn in preparation for the exclusive focus on literary reading and thinking which follows in Part II.

*

For Bion, thought is not 'a product of thinking'. Rather, 'thinking is a development forced on the psyche by the pressure of thoughts and not the other way round'. Thinking, then, is an 'apparatus' that 'has to be called into existence to cope with thoughts'.[41] Thoughts are the raw, primitive, inchoate sense-impressions related to emotional experience. Bion called these 'beta elements', and the thinking apparatus that processes and converts the 'beta' sense-data, he called 'alpha function'.[42] The most elemental of thoughts is when the infant's expectation of a breast meets not with 'an emotional experience of satisfaction' but with 'frustration'. Unable to process the experience by itself, the infant has to 'evacuate these elements into the mother, relying on her to do whatever has to be done to convert them into a form suitable for employment as alpha-elements'.[43] The mother transforms – or to use another key concept for Bion, 'contains'[44] – the emotional experience (beta elements) that the infant is unable to bear and converts and makes them available to the infant in bearable form (as alpha elements). When the infant's 'capacity for toleration of frustration is sufficient the "no breast" inside becomes a thought, and an apparatus for "thinking" it [alpha function] develops'. However, if the infant's feeling state is not accepted or borne by the mother, it is 'imposed' instead on the infant's rudimentary consciousness, which 'cannot carry the burden placed on it'. The unprocessed feeling state is internalized, not as a fearful experience made tolerable, but as 'a nameless dread'.[45] These untransformed beta elements are then liable to be discharged through 'mindless actions' or, alternatively, 'evacuated into the body, resulting in somatic symptoms or illnesses'.[46] The following account from Karen Horney's clinical experience pinpoints the affinity between Bion's theory of thinking and the phenomenon now known as alexithymia, as well as the relation of both to physical pain. 'The more remote a person is from their inner life, the less alive they are':

> The unavailability [and] unawareness of inner experiences gives a person a feeling of emptiness or nothingness, which in itself may or may not be conscious. But whether this feeling is conscious or not, it is in any case frightening. On the grounds of our clinical experiences we can understand those philosophers who contend that anxiety ultimately is the fear of nothingness (Kierkegaard) or the fear of nonbeing (Tillich). . . . This dread of nothingness may appear in rather direct forms, such as a gnawing and painful feeling of bodily emptiness [or] in the attempts to run away from it.[47]

Nameless dread, the engulfing terror of abandonment and annihilation, 'rather than stimulating the psychic work needed to produce mental representations . . . provoke[s] a wound in the mind . . . a haemorrhage of representation, a pain with no image . . . a blank slate . . . a hole'.[48] Emotional states which are thus unable to be converted or released through commensurate mental realization become painfully *contained* by the body instead. For Bion, it is this catastrophic 'breakdown in the development of the apparatus for "thinking" or dealing with thoughts, [that] the psychoanalytic situation addresses'.[49]

As is widely acknowledged, this is a critical re-writing of the purpose of psychoanalysis. Indeed, as Thomas Ogden points out, Bion's speculations about psychological events in the mother-infant relationship are 'merely metaphors . . . for what occurs at an unconscious level in the analytic relationship'.[50] The latter was, says Howard Levine, 'the true north of psychoanalytic inquiry', for Bion, who 'regarded anything else as *hearsay evidence*'.[51] The role of the analyst is not only to uncover and resolve hidden or unconscious conflict but to build and strengthen the very capacity for mental representation: to make thinkable previously inchoate proto-thoughts by allowing them to be realized in verbalized form.[52] Accordingly, the goals of contemporary psychoanalysis aim 'primarily at the expansion of the mental container'[53] for emotional experience. 'The idea of the container-contained addresses not what we think, but the way we think . . . how we process lived experience and what occurs psychically when we are unable to do psychological work with that experience.'[54] It is not that people are without containers for experience, but rather that the latter are often inadequate.

> One often discovers that the very means by which [patients] have forestalled the real or imagined threats of catastrophic abandonment, annihilation anxiety and nameless dread – that is, the defensive organizations that allow a part of their psyches to achieve some degree of . . . regulation

and development – are responsible for the distress that brings them to treatment.[55]

In other words, the container employed is effectively a defence against emotional reality rather than a means to think it, and the meaning thereby contained is itself empty, a husk. What is required of the psychoanalyst is 'to lend his or her transformative capacities to the patient',[56] to endure or host whatever thought they cannot bear to think, giving 'form to this amorphous mass by endowing it with a place in space and a moment in time'.[57] This, I will suggest in Part II, is where reading, too, can lend its transformative power, catalysing, through the emotional resonances generated in the here and now encounter with a literary text, a viable thought, a vital meaning, out of the previously inadmissible and unsayable.

The turn to Bion, here at the close of Part I, brings me full circle to my starting-point in relation to reading and pain which, as outlined in the Preface, started with a study of reading and depression. That work began from the Bion-inspired intuition that literature might be an analogue and adjunct to psychoanalysis in helping people to think about their experience. This seemed an especially urgent task given not only the prevalence of depressive symptoms in the Western world but in view of Bion's proposal that, even in the healthy psyche, the apparatus for thinking is a late evolutionary development which, as a means to manage the complex and unruly emotional data given off by the 'demands of reality', is seriously underdeveloped.[58] Thinking needs all the help it can get. For truth, as Bion insisted, is 'as essential for emotional growth as food is for the body: without it the mind dies of starvation'.[59] Bion's wonted physical simile ('the welfare of the patient demands a constant supply of truth as inevitably as his physical survival demands food'[60]) is especially compelling and resonant as I turn to consider the emotional power of literature in relation to the experience of chronic bodily pain.

I do so armed with an understanding of chronic pain, offered in the foregoing chapters, which, as explained in the Preface, I did not have when I first embarked on this work. In Part II, I will draw on much of the thinking introduced here, as well as seek to align it with current theories around reading and psychology and reading and mental health. The chief function of Part I, however, has been to provide a bedrock or landscape in which to situate what is a small and vulnerable though (to me) powerful experiment in reading and pain.

'In reading'
Chronic pain, literature, therapy

5

Why reading? Starting points and key concepts

Part II is the heart of this book. It is based on primary evidence of the value of reading literature for people living with chronic pain, as demonstrated by a study carried out by a multidisciplinary research team at the University of Liverpool in a pain clinic in North West England. The immediate context for this research, as we shall see, is a body of work which has grown up over the past two decades or so around the phenomenon of shared group reading. The origins of the specific model of shared reading in question, however, could hardly have been farther from the context of clinically diagnosed chronic pain in which this chapter finds and places it.

In the late 1990s, a group of extra-mural teachers of English Literature set up a reading group in one of the most disadvantaged areas of Merseyside. It was a reading group with a difference. Books were not read in advance, as in conventional book clubs, nor was the reading material confined to contemporary fiction. Instead, fiction and poetry from across the ages were read aloud together. As the demand for groups grew, the charity, The Reader, was founded, and with it an international movement.[1] When members of the growing number of groups consistently reported improved wellbeing as a result of their experience of shared reading, health care providers became interested in commissioning the groups as part of their care programmes. But such commissions required robust evidence of the impact on health. This demand initiated a series of well-documented studies based in prisons,[2] GP surgeries,[3] care homes[4] and community contexts,[5] which, carried out with psychologists and medical experts and using standard measures of quality of life and psychological health and wellbeing, found alleviation in the symptoms of a range of mental health conditions.

The notion of literary reading for health is by no means a twenty-first-century phenomenon. On the contrary, a theoretical rationale for these studies was already established in the fields of classical poetics, philosophy and psychoanalysis, as well as literary studies.[6] Nonetheless, this was arguably the first sustained body of work to pursue systematically the claims that the reading of literature per se – as distinct from reading as a programmatic intervention, such as in bibliotherapy – had the power to heal.[7]

Building as it did (and as I have described in the Preface) on these antecedent studies, the literary reading and chronic pain study was duly scientific in orientation. We set out to compare the relative impact on the (reported) experience of physical pain and psychological wellbeing (emotion and mood in particular) of engaging in group CBT and group Shared Reading. This suited both the 'reading' researchers who had long sought to assess the value of literary reading alongside a formal therapeutic programme, and, as we saw in Chapter 1, CBT is the standard psychosocial intervention in relation to chronic pain (as it is for many diagnosed conditions). It also matched the care agenda of the pain consultants who invited the study, and who were all too conscious that a six-week course of therapy was woefully inadequate for meeting the needs of their patients who in many cases *keep coming back for years and years*. The emphasis in pain treatment, they explained, is *a switch from a therapeutic cure, which you know does not exist, to providing support over a long period of time and trying to help people get through their setbacks and flare-ups. Don't forget, these are people who have been around hospital doctors and primary care an awful lot. They know that there's no point in going to Accident & Emergency. There's no point in going to see the GP. So their point of contact with any support is very often us and only us.* In a situation in which patients needed as much support as they could possibly get, therefore, the goal was never to assert the value of one group experience over another – CBT bad, Shared Reading good, for example. Rather, the purpose was to identify the distinctive benefits of each intervention with a view to their being not alternatives but adjuncts to one another as part of a pain management package. The pain consultants again: *You have to be realistic about what you may achieve. You're not going to cure anybody, so you need to have the mindset that you are doing the best for the patient and that the patient will appreciate you're doing the best you can. It's important that they feel better than they would do if you weren't doing what you are doing.*[8]

To describe the study in brief.[9]

Following ethical approval by a UK National Health Service Research Ethics Committee, a five-week CBT group (the standard duration, more or less, for CBT in NHS contexts) and a twenty-two-week Shared Reading group (in line with the optimum minimum length recommended by previous research studies) were set up to run in parallel for chronic pain patients at the hospital where they attended their routine pain clinic. CBT group members joined the Shared Reading group after the completion of the CBT course. As we shall see, the groups were made up of a mix of genders, ages (roughly ranging from people in their twenties to those in their seventies) and backgrounds. As the consultants pointed out, however, many *are from an inner city environment and most of them – the vast majority – are living on benefits, and they've had a continuous assault on their living standards for many years. They're constantly having to go through assessments to ascertain their eligibility for state benefits. That adds an extra layer of complexity to the condition, and to our therapeutic relationship with them; sometimes people are frightened to report an improvement because it might have a financial consequence.*

Participants completed the Positive and Negative Affect Scale (PANAS) immediately following each CBT and Shared Reading session.[10] This standardized scale is one of the most widely used for assessing emotion and mood and consists of words describing emotions – ten positive (e.g. 'enthusiastic', 'excited') and ten negative (e.g. 'nervous', 'afraid'), and asks participants to write next to each word the extent to which they are feeling each emotion on a scale of 1–5 (1 = not at all; 5 = extremely). In addition, participants in our study were asked to write down two words or phrases which best described their experience on that occasion. All participants also kept twice-daily (twelve-hourly) pain and emotion diaries. Pain severity was recorded using a 0–10 rating scale (0 = non-existent, 10 = severe) at twelve-hour intervals, and participants wrote down two words to describe their feelings, using as a guide (but not restricted to) those listed on the PANAS.

Although the sample size was small, the data generated by twice-daily participant reports over six months was considerable and sufficient to offer demonstration of perceptible trends and statistically significant improvements in chronic pain and mood for participants after engaging in Shared Reading (see Tables 1 and 2 below). These included a strongly significant correlation between high scores for pain severity and low (negative) scores for emotion. They also showed that pain ratings after the weekly Shared Reading session were lower than the overall mean, and lower than two days before and two days after the reading group session. Pain ratings two days after Shared Reading were also lower than two days before the reading group, suggesting the possibility of some prolonged effect beyond the duration of the group itself. The emotion rating was also higher on the evening following the Shared Reading group than two days before or two days after. The scores for CBT, by contrast, showed a pain score above the overall mean and an emotion score below the overall mean. Although the emotion score was higher after the session than either two days before or two days after, there is considerably less evidence here that CBT affected pain and emotion beyond the duration of the group.

These statistics seem startlingly consistent when baldly stated. They were less surprising to those of us who, as part of the qualitative research

Table 1 Pain and Emotion Ratings before and after Attendances at Shared Reading Sessions

	Pain Rating 0–10		Emotion (±- scale, 1–9)	
Overall (24/7)	Mean: 6.00	Valid N: 1665	Mean: 3.96	Valid N: 1573
Evening, two days before	Mean: 6.51	Valid N: 81	Mean: 4.07	Valid N: 76
Evening, Shared Reading Session	Mean: 5.69	Valid N: 78	Mean: 4.69	Valid N: 78
Evening, two days after	Mean: 6.31	Valid N: 92	Mean: 3.99	Valid N: 84

Table 2 Pain and Emotion Ratings before and after Attendances at CBT Sessions

	Pain Rating 0–10		Emotion (± scale, 1–9)	
Overall (24/7)	Mean: 6.00	Valid N: 1665	Mean: 3.96	Valid N: 1573
Evening, two days before	Mean: 7.55	Valid N: 11	Mean: 2.3	Valid N: 10
Evening, CBT session	Mean: 7.59	Valid N: 11	Mean: 3.5	Valid N: 10
Evening, two days after	Mean: 7.59	Valid N: 11	Mean: 2.4	Valid N: 10

in this mixed-methods study, subsequently interviewed all participants. The dual finding of higher emotion and lower pain scores after the reading group correlated with participants frequently stating, for example, that they enjoyed a better night's sleep on the evening of the Shared Reading session. As a multidisciplinary research team, we also *saw* the contrastive experience of CBT and Shared Reading. Sessions were video- and audio-recorded for analysis by the combined expertise of specialists in linguistics, psychology, occupational therapy and literary studies. For this purpose, we adopted the innovative method developed and refined in preceding studies of Shared Reading, which concentrates on moments of 'live "happening"', where 'the literature seems to get through to participants and itself to come alive through them',[11] and which uses, for reliable identification of these instances, a rating system (0–5 where 5 = 'hot/live', 0 = 'cold/dead') based on William James's description of 'emotional excitement'. 'There are dead feelings, dead ideas, and cold beliefs, and there are hot and live ones; and when one grows hot and alive within us, everything has to re-crystallize about it. These hot parts are the centres of our dynamic energy, whereas the cold parts leave us indifferent and passive in proportion to their coldness.'[12] The case studies which follow coalesce around hot/live instances identified in this way. As we shall see, the video-recordings and interviews not only helped to corroborate *that* the reading was beneficial for these pain patients. They were richly suggestive of *how* it was so, the process by which reading alleviated perceived pain. And the 'how' was sometimes counter-intuitive. For example, one key finding which emerged from collating the data from the post-session questionnaires and the evidence from the video-recordings and interviews was that 'feeling good' after Shared Reading did not routinely coincide with the experience of exclusively positive emotion within the Shared Reading session. Indeed, it was quite typical for participants to note, for example, 'Some sadness but feeling better, less pain', or 'My emotions are sad, a bit down, but glad; mixed emotions'; or to feel energized by the reading despite the pain suffered: 'Inspiring and good interaction. Suffered from back pain most of this session a little'; 'Very sore; enjoying the book'. This complexity was matched, as we shall see, by the wider range and intensity of emotions both reported and witnessed in Shared Reading as compared to CBT.

This richness has propelled me to return to this material for the present book, to go beyond establishing dominant themes (which are already published and which, as appropriate, I will rehearse again here) in order to 'piece out' individualized, nuanced and granular case studies of participants' comparative experiences of Shared Reading and CBT.

A few further preliminaries are necessary to set the scene, however.

The psychology of reading

As outlined above, the body of work which has grown up around reading and health at Liverpool originated outside of a research agenda of any kind, let alone a health-oriented one: it started with a book and a group of people in a library, no more. One consequence is that the relationship of this work to the (highly relevant) scientific study of literature and the psychology of reading, which was taking place over roughly the same time period (since the 1990s) in Europe and North America, has been, until relatively recently, piecemeal, unplanned and partial, though always fruitful.[13] In this section, as part of my backfill project of drawing on a range of discourses to try to understand 'why literary reading?' for chronic pain, I seek to bring together corroborative insights from these two separately developed areas of exploration.

The aspects from the field of reading psychology and scientific-empirical studies of reading which bear most directly on reading and health are the roles of, on the one hand, emotion and empathy, and on the other, the formal properties of literary texts in prompting transformative reading experiences. In what follows, I explain and illustrate these ideas with reference to transcripts of two video-recorded sessions from the chronic pain reading group. In one sense, these exemplary sessions act as a kind of template to highlight already rigorously researched elements of literary reading, which are present across all the examples encountered in this chapter, and whose influence we can take for granted as being always there and, more or less, strong. At the same time, these instances give an early sense of the rich potential for Shared Reading to demonstrate, in a natural setting, phenomena that have hitherto, or until very recently, been studied almost exclusively in laboratory conditions. Above all, these initial examples introduce the reader to Shared Reading as a form and a happening, in advance of the individualized case studies which ensue.

Emotion and empathy

The clear consensus which has emerged over the last three decades among scholars of reading is that literature is an affective context. This emphasis was initiated in part by the countermovement to the postmodernist sensibility which had dominated literary studies within the final quarter of the twentieth century and which had held that literature, like any text, was merely a linguistic system of signs with no special claims or value within culture. As Terry Eagleton put it, 'anything can be literature' or 'can cease to be literature'[14] according to the endorsement or otherwise of prevailing ideologies. Resistance to *this* 'specialized ideology' – in the service of which literary scholars 'produced readings of texts and elaborations of literary theory in an institutional culture [inhabited] almost exclusively by fellow scholars and senior students'[15] – coincided with a new interest, among researchers in literature, language, aesthetics and psychology,[16] in the real (as opposed to the assumed or ideal) reader: 'the ordinary reader, who . . . continues to read for the pleasure of [exploring] the world of the text, rather than for the development of a deconstructionist or historicist perspective'.[17] As the early pioneers in this new field of empirical literary studies ventured that 'feeling is the primary vehicle'[18] for such exploration, so, in the now substantial field of readerly 'absorption',[19] 'emotional engagement'[20] is widely recognized to be the strongest mediator of deep involvement with a literary text. Our own research is highly corroborative of these conclusions and frequently attests to the suddenness, involuntariness and neo-physical quality of the emotional response.[21]

So to start with this basic element of 'real' reading, and to give a flavour of the kind of emotional involvement literature compels, here are some excerpts from a Shared Reading session within our study which took place around halfway through the programme as a whole (week 13 of 22). The session scored neither highest nor lowest on the PANAS, so it might be thought of as representative. But the session also proved (both at the interview and in later reading sessions) to be an important touchstone for group members and for the group leader and thus will be so for the ensuing chapters also. The words used by group members to describe their mood immediately after the session were uniform in their register and unusually intense: 'very emotional, but relaxed'; 'feeling good'; 'energized; happy'; 'very emotional; very good session'.

*　　*　　*

The group gathers on the same day every week in a meeting room within the city centre hospital, where the group members routinely attend the pain clinic. The regular tables and chairs have been rearranged to form a square at the centre. The group leader, one of the original founders of The Reader, is also a long-time chronic pain sufferer and a wheelchair user. As is customary in Shared Reading, she begins the session formally (as group members share a hot drink and snacks) by distributing the text in paper form to all members, then proceeds to read the text aloud to the group.

A note on the reading material. Each ninety-minute Shared Reading session combines fiction (which is read and discussed during the first hour) and poetry (which concludes the meeting). The selection of texts – especially of longer fictional works with which the group might live for weeks – is customarily made on the basis of reading 'tasters' (usually up to six possible choices) and then on group consensus as to preference. In a pilot version of the chronic pain study, the group leader's instinct of using shorter fiction and poetry was vindicated. Shorter texts catered for potential impairment of concentration, through tiredness, analgesic or antidepressant medication, or from sitting for any length of time (participants sometimes felt it necessary to stand up and walk around). They also made the sessions 'stand-alone' in nature, thus minimizing the impact of intermittent attendance, given the significant obstacles for participants of walking long distances and accessing public transport. The group leader's choice to begin with lighter reading fare and progress to more difficult literature needed to be quickly revised, however. From the outset, all group members showed a strong preference for emotionally and intellectually demanding and complex material.[22] On the basis of this experience, the chronic pain study proper selected a mix of (mostly

English and American) poetry and shorter fiction from the nineteenth century to the present day.

This week the group is reading Edith Wharton's short story 'Mrs Manstey's View', in which the protagonist, a widow, lives in the back room on the third floor of a New York boarding house, with a view from her window which is not 'striking', but is to her 'full of beauty and interest'. Though increasingly alone – through infirmity and distance from her only (married) child – Mrs Manstey has 'long since accepted as a matter of course her solitary life'. The group leader reads:

> Mrs Manstey had never been a sociable woman and during her husband's lifetime his companionship had been all-sufficient to her. For many years she had cherished a desire to live in the country, to have a hen-house and a garden, but this longing had faded with age, leaving only in the breast of the uncommunicative old woman a vague tenderness for plants and animals. It was, perhaps, this tenderness which made her cling so fervently to her view from her window, a view in which the most optimistic eye would at first have failed to discover anything admirable. . . . Perhaps at heart Mrs Manstey was an artist. At all events she was sensible of many changes of colour unnoticed by the average eye and dear to her as the green of early spring was the black lattice of branches against a cold sulphur sky at the close of a snowy day. . . . The view surrounded and shaped her life as the sea does a lonely island. . . . Mrs Manstey's real friends were the denizens of the yards, the hyacinths, the magnolia, the green parrot, the maid who fed the cats, the doctor who studied late behind his mustard-coloured curtains, and the confidant of her tenderer musings was the church-spire floating in the sunset.[23]

Here is an edited and abbreviated version of the ensuing discussion.

> *Eve: Ah, poor woman. She's living life through everyone else. That's to do with her age and her disability. But it's not a life is it. It's restrictive, I think.*
>
> *Fay: You mean it's just – an existence. It says she's clinging to the view.*
>
> *Deborah: She's really cocooned herself. The daughter left, the husband passed – No-one else can leave. There's no threat. She connects with the world by watching and takes comfort in people's habits and their processes. It's a very sort of secure connection – a safe connection.*
>
> *June: This upsets me, you know, 'cause my dad can't, my dad doesn't go out. But he knows the people going to church, and says Mrs So and So passes every day. It quite upsets me thinking – Is that all there is for him? That he's content like that?*

David now notices how words of affection – 'cherished', 'tenderness', 'longing' – are attached not to people but to the natural world – 'hen-house and garden', 'plants and animals'.

> *David: She seems to me quite – quite happy. The window is her friend and the environment beyond the window. It's her life. The garden and what she can see out of her window.*
> *Fay: You mean she's actually happier in the window. The garden's alive, it's growing.*
> *June: Yes [reading], 'The confidant of her tenderer musings was the church spire floating in the sunset'. Isn't that lovely? You can imagine that lovely scene.*
> *John: [pointing to and reading the sentence 'she was sensible of many changes of colour unnoticed by the average eye'] She even notices things in tiny detail that we wouldn't – they'd bypass us.*
> *Deborah: She's taking pleasure out of the little things that we take for granted when we're rushing past and you're full of everything.*
> *Eve: Not seeing what's just around us, normal things.*

The central event of the story is when Mrs Manstey receives the news that a neighbour plans to build an extension – 'right back to the end of the yard [and] right up to the roof' – obscuring the view from the window. 'Soon the wisteria would bloom, then the horse-chestnut, but not for her. Between her eyes and them a barrier of brick and mortar would swiftly rise; presently even the spire would disappear and all her radiant world be blotted out.'[24] There are gasps and looks of astonishment from the group members.

> *Fay: Ahhh that's sad. She's going to feel it's closing her in.*
> *David: She's like a poor woman whose whole world is collapsing. Her world will end. She's going to lose everything.*
> *June: It's like someone just pulled the blind down. 'All that radiant world' – 'even the spire would disappear'. How often do you see a radiant world when you're wandering around? really you know really? how do you get to see a radiant world?*

*   *   *

'Compared to non-literary narratives, literary narratives amplify and "flesh out" . . . affective and embodied re-presentations . . . transport[ing] a reader from the everyday world to the vividly imagined world of the text.'[25] 'Objects, people, and places in the imaginal world of the text are given a multimodal sensuous presence, constituting a vividly imagined "other".[26] Frequently in Shared Reading, the sense of 'fleshed out' reality is so powerful as to reach directly into the affective real life of the reader. *It upsets me, Aah, that's sad* are not mere formal expressions of sentiment but rather the vocal sign that emotions are the carriers of the affective life of the book into the embodied life of the reader. 'Feeling, as a form of incipient thinking struggling for articulation, is the primary experience without which in the first place, nothing to felt purpose follows in the second.'[27]

One 'purpose' and value of reading, from a psychological point of view, is to increase empathy and, thereby, theory of mind, the psychological term for the capacity (as we saw in Part I) to mentalize or better understand ourselves and others. When June thinks instinctively of her own father, she is, according to the Canadian psychologist Keith Oatley, in *Such Stuff as Dreams: The Psychology of Fiction*, doing something essential to the process of reading fiction: 'When we understand an action as we read about it in a novel, our understanding depends on making a version of the action ourselves inwardly.'[28] Oatley likens what happens in fiction reading, at the micro level, to the phenomenon of mirror neurons, where the same neurons fire when a task is performed as when it is perceived to be performed. At the macro level, he describes fiction as 'the mind's flight simulator'.[29] Through extensive psychological experiments, Oatley and his colleagues have demonstrated that literary narratives offer readers immersive simulative models of the social world, and social interactions, which facilitate understanding of others who are different from ourselves, and which augment the capacity for empathy and social inference. Previous Shared Reading studies have likewise found that the internalization of alternative behaviours through absorption with fictional scenarios of action and reaction,[30] and practice in understanding from a range of imagined positions and viewpoints,[31] encourages mental-emotional agility[32] and stimulates 'metacognition and high-level mentalisation in relation to deepened and expanded emotional investment in human pursuits (created by the text)'.[33]

The 'flight' which we see the group members imaginatively make in reading together 'Mrs Manstey's View' has several mentalizing 'pay-offs', so to speak. The first relates to the protagonist's situation, which at first – and intermittently throughout the session – appears unhealthily limiting: *Just – an existence . . . very restrictive, There's no threat.* The sense that Mrs Manstey is simply seeking, more or less, to survive her life and the tendency to see her as 'clinging' to the view from her window as a mode of self-protection (*She's really cocooned herself*, the view is *comfort*), is subtly modulated as the session goes on. What Deborah calls a *secure [and] safe connection* becomes something more admirable and distinctive, not merely defensive. John's recognition of Mrs Manstey 'the artist', noticing what would bypass the 'average' eye,[34] and June's wondering question (*How often do you see a radiant world?*) are picked up by Deborah and Eve as they recall this moment in the story, where Mrs Manstey is visited by her landlady (the only occasion on which we witness Mrs Manstey with human companionship) and remarks that the magnolia is out earlier than usual this year. '"The what?"' enquires the landlady. '"I didn't know there was a magnolia there."'[35]

> *Eve: It's like the landlady gets on with life but she's blinkered. She doesn't see what's going on around.*
> *Deborah: And she doesn't see what's important to Mrs Manstey.*

What is significant here is the group members' own seeing of something that counts as an achievement in Mrs Manstey, when weighed against the landlady's double failure of vision, in respect of 'what's important' both in the view and to Mrs Manstey. Where the group began by seeing Mrs Manstey's situation as primarily restrictive and as a function (to be regretted) of her disability, this later feat of discrimination is the outcome of their inhabiting 'Mrs Manstey's View' – her perspective, her mindset – as the landlady cannot, and as no person easily could without the help of the story. The story exists, indeed, to provoke these inversions and reversals and re-perspectivizing, from outward to inward and back again. It does not demand that these readers make any literal or conscious connection with the disabling limitation of their own lives; yet it implicitly arouses such imaginative recognitions even so. This is Oatley's point of course, his rationale for why we need literary narrative. 'Fiction', says Oatley, 'is not just a slice of life, not just entertainment, not just escape from the everyday. [It offers] a model that we as readers construct in collaboration with the writer, which can enable us to see others and ourselves more clearly'.[36] These active mental models extend the reader's repertoire of emotion, experience and empathy and, as one Shared Reading study put it, offer 'a testing ground for new ways of being'.[37] That the readers we have witnessed are active in emotionally and imaginatively immersed collaboration with *one another* as well as with the text is an important phenomenon to which I return at the close of this section of the book.

Foregrounding and felt sense

For David Miall and Donald Kuiken, with whose model of affective reading the ensuing chapters will be frequently in dialogue, the kind of feelings we have seen summoned by literary reading can be traced to what is known in literary and linguistic theory as *foregrounding*. The term refers to the stylistic variations which occur at levels of sound (rhythm, rhyme, alliteration), grammar (syntactic irregularity, high patterning) and semantics (imagery, irony).

Drawing on the thinking of twentieth-century literary and aesthetic theorist Jan Mukařovský, who originated the term, 'the purpose of foregrounding', say Miall and Kuiken, 'is to disrupt everyday communication . . . present[ing] meanings with an intricacy and complexity that ordinary language does not normally allow'.[38] 'Foregrounding is the opposite of automatization, that is, the deautomatization of an act; the more an act is automatized, the less it is consciously executed; the more it is foregrounded, the more completely conscious does it become. Objectively speaking: automatization schematizes an event; foregrounding means the violation of the scheme.'[39] Miall and Kuiken point out the close relation between the process of deautomatization as described by Mukařovský and the concept of *defamiliarization* or *making strange* introduced by the Russian formalist school of literary criticism in the early decades of the twentieth century. 'Art exists', wrote Victor Shklovsky, 'that one may recover the sensation of life; it exists to make one feel things. . . . The purpose of art is to impart the sensation of things as they are perceived and not as they are known . . . to make objects "unfamiliar", to make forms difficult, to increase the difficulty and length of perception'.[40] Miall and Kuiken and their colleagues have proposed and tested across multiple studies the psychological process elicited in the reader by foregrounding: 'When perception has been deautomatized, a reader employs the feelings that have been evoked to find or create a context in which the defamiliarized aspects of the story can be located', or 'refamiliarized'.[41] In brief, foregrounding is the affective catalyst to the re-visioning of perspective, literally seeing things again, anew, differently. Correspondingly, in Shared Reading, the challenging depth and difficulty of the literary language (the very aspect which the chronic pain group instinctively preferred and sought) have been found to block automatic responses and speech behaviours, thereby creating access and slowed deep thinking in relation to areas of experience for which no ready language exists.[42]

Let me illustrate the defamiliarizing-refamiliarizing process as Miall and Kuiken describe it by reference to the 'purest' version of it I could find from the Shared Reading sessions with the chronic pain group. The session occurred relatively early in the programme (session 6) when the group's exposure to poetry was still fairly limited and this encounter with Modernist poet Maria Rainer Rilke's work was by far the most 'difficult' to date.

* * *

Group Leader: The poem is called 'Evening'. [Reads the poem, three short stanzas, in full.[43]]
June: It's a different one, a hard one.

Eve: I can see him putting on the 'darkening blue coat'. If you are ever standing, when it's going dark, and [slowly moving palms together, one over the other] the light's moving up to meet it and there's a blurred bit in the middle, a fine line, before the darkness falls [hand sweeps downwards] and it never seems to go fully dark. There's always that blurred bit in between.

Group Leader: That's a lovely way of describing it.

June: It makes me think of years ago when people used to close curtains because of a death.

David: It's not a morbid poem though.

Deborah: No, because it's full of – life or – movement.

The group leader re-reads the poem's first two stanzas.

Susan: 'Not at home in either one' – either one what?

Deborah: That middle stanza is all about everything that isn't – 'not quite so still', 'not calling to eternity'. It doesn't say 'it's not this but it is that' – just 'it isn't', 'it's not'.

Susan: It's like – limbo isn't it?

June: [reverting to the final line of stanza one] Yes, it says 'One journeying to heaven, one that falls' – falls where?.

Presently, the group leader re-reads the final stanza, which closes with 'alternately stone in you and star':

Group Leader: What is 'stone in you'? If I said 'I've got stone in me' – what would that mean?

Fay: Stone is a – heaviness – as opposed to the lightness of the star. I think of having a heavy feeling on you, when all of a sudden it lifts and you get that – ah – you can breathe.

Susan: I wonder though – maybe – if you've got stone in you, are you grounded?

Group Leader: So the stone isn't necessarily all bad? It's – earthed?

David: It can go either way, at any point. 'Now bounded, now immeasurable'. It's ups and downs, going in and out of both.

June: Is it that we're always moving between them? Two different states – not stuck in either one of them.

Susan: It's both together – 'stone in you and star'.

June: 'Falls' . . . 'and rises'.

Fay: If you look at the darkening at evening, like Eve says, while the sky comes down, it does look like the earth is moving up as well.

Deborah: I wonder – is that why it's called 'Evening', not 'Night'?

I identify three key elements from Miall's and Kuiken's account of foregrounding and affect. Firstly, is increased reading time. Readers 'dwell on'[44] foregrounded elements, 'slow their reading and report greater uncertainty. . . . It is these moments that especially challenge the reader's existing framework for understanding [and] may motivate attempts to revise and reconstruct [their] interpretive framework'.[45] If anything, encountering foregrounded features in the context of Shared Reading 'slows' the reading further as group members hold in common their uncertainty and grapple with it cooperatively (*either one what?; falls where?; what is stone in you?*).

Secondly, reading motivates 'an attentional pause' wherein the reader may 'review the textual context in order to discern, delimit, or develop the novel meanings suggested by the foregrounded passage'.[46] June, for example, at her first utterance, looks back more attentively at stanza one, pauses at 'one that falls' on realizing that the poem supplies no tidy opposite to 'heaven', and thence, in her final utterance (*Falls . . . and rises*), herself foregrounds how 'falls' at the end of stanza one is opposed to 'rises' at the end of stanza two.

Thirdly, 'feeling struck, captured, held, in response to foregrounding . . . heightens feeling tone'[47] and 'sensitize[s] the reader to other passages having similar affective connotations', in a process of 'reattentional activity'[48] or refamiliarization. A stunning example is Deborah's sudden recognition of the affective resonance of the title 'Evening', one that is first picked up, in fact, by Eve's expressive description of the *fine line . . . in between* light and dark, and remembered by Fay at the end of the discussion. Striking, too, is that final movement of the discussion, where the meaning and designation of the 'state' figured in the poem are held in fluid, mobile suspension, as the group's response effectively recreates the indefiniteness of the poem: *It can go either way, at any point . . . ups and downs, . . . in and out . . . moving between . . . not stuck in either . . . both together.* It is as if the group is occupying that *not* or *isn't* space which Deborah locates in stanza two – *It's about everything that isn't.* This very formulation is a linguistic trace of the disruption to 'everyday' default responses impelled by the literary text as it generates refreshed language and thinking in place of familiar automaticity.

Indeed, I thus slow down and explicate the processes involved not merely to show the applicability of the concept of defamiliarization in this context, but chiefly to illustrate how the difficulty and unfamiliarity of the poem's language obstruct easy facility and dislodge reliance on an automatic discourse and mindset. This is a critical element in literature's power to evoke what Miall and Kuiken call 'self-modifying feelings', wherein existing personal thoughts and feelings are confronted, realized or experienced in a new form, and recontextualized or reconfigured in an 'altered understanding of the reader's own lifeworld'.[49] 'Such feelings are likely to be subtle and fugitive rather than named' and always dependent upon 'how compelling are the emotional qualities of the text, and what personal concerns, memories and experiences a reader brings'.[50] In advance of the extended examples of this process which absorb the coming chapters, I offer here a tiny glimpse of such a fugitive shift. At one point, June suggests, in response to Susan and Fay alike, that the group's common chronic condition left them all too *grounded and heavy most of the time.* The group leader ventured, *You must have some star?* June responded, thoughtfully *I do.* The group then exchanged, with evident enjoyment, their personal 'star' – seeing grandchildren, watching their favourite football team, walking the dog, sharing music with friends. The group is by this stage so cognitively and affectively immersed – so 'at home' – in the de-automatizing terms of the poem, that the group leader has only to re-mobilize one of the poem's central metaphors to re-energize and propel the talk in a non-default direction. As we shall see, this brake on a tendency towards defeatism, and the provision of an alternative language for painful experience, was one key contrast between the emotional tone of Shared Reading as compared with CBT.

One danger of slowing down the reading process in this way, however, is that the quick and 'subtle' vitality of these moments – their galvanic and sudden emergence – can be lost. More often than not, as will be richly demonstrated in the chapters which follow, reappraisal of even far past experience is 'an amalgam of old, long-felt content and a sudden new perspective, which the poem tacitly calls for'.[51] In Shared Reading, emotions reclaim their evolutionary value by being 'restored to urgent messages of feeling that usefully tell of a now more internal fact, a psychological reality which . . . should not be ignored'.[52] This is where the work of Eugene Gendlin, which has provided a philosophical foundation for Kuiken et al.'s theory of self-modifying feelings, is an especially useful corrective.

Gendlin was a philosopher of experience and process, influenced by thinkers in the phenomenological tradition (Husserl, Heidegger, Merleau-Ponty, among others). He explored the relation of implicit to explicit knowing, of experience to conceptual meaning and the formulating process from one to another. 'I use the word "experiencing" to denote *concrete* experience . . . the *raw*, present, ongoing *functioning* (in us) of what is usually called experience.' 'Experiencing is an aspect of human living that is constant, like body life, metabolism, sensory input. . . . [the] ever present, underlying phenomenon of inwardly sentient living.' Another term for experiencing is 'felt meaning'. Meaning involves 'a powerful *felt* dimension of experience that is pre-logical and that functions importantly in what we think. . . . Felt meaning functions as the experienced side of all thought'. What is required in the translation from implicit experience to explicit concept is to 'think with the intricacy of situations'. Yet it is equally the case that in the very process of such formulation it will be found that 'the experiential side always exceeds the concepts. . . . There is always . . . an implicit experiential context that is *more* than any formed form'.[53] That is to say, we can only ever put a few aspects of felt meaning into words. Gendlin more than once uses the example of a poet in the midst of composition:

> How does the poet recognize the right line when it comes? . . . The poet rejected the many lines because the more precise implying *continued to hang there*. None of those lines could *take it along*. Now it *no longer hangs there*, because that special line has *carried the implying forward*.[54]

For Kuiken et al., it is as if the reading process is analogous to, or the other 'side' of, the writing process as Gendlin describes it. 'Embodied and dynamic participation' in a literary text produces 'the felt sense of something "more" than is accessible through habitual preconceptions'. This motivates absorbed, receptive attention to 'uncovering' the 'more', and thence leads to a 'felt shift' in perception, an 'altered sense', something 'freshly realized'.[55] Kuiken calls this 'expressive enactment'.[56] In the blurring of boundaries between self and text – such that a figure in the text might be 'brought to presence, as in method acting' – an affective resonance is created which (in Gendlin's terms) 'carries forward, rather than merely matches and externalises',[57] an existing perspective. I will unpack the event of expressive enactment more fully in the next chapter. But as an interim shorthand approximation to this process, take the group's volte-face at the close of 'Mrs Manstey's View', when, seriously ill, the protagonist is carried to the window by her nurse:

> It was hard for Mrs Manstey to breathe. Each moment it grew more difficult. . . . But the view at least was there. The spire was golden now. . . .
>
> Mrs Manstey's head fell back and smiling, she died.
>
> That day the building of the extension was resumed.[58]
>
> *Deborah: For her the building had stopped, for her it never happened.*
>
> *Fay: It was still there when she died. Her world was still there. I think that's lovely.*

The notion of the view being *still there* is not belittled or dismissed as illusory, as the group member's 'habitual preconception' would have dictated at the opening of the story. Rather, it is newly valued as Mrs Manstey's 'felt meaning', her very last, and the only one that matters here and now.

Gendlin's philosophy is especially useful to this book because it is not theoretical only but personalized and practical. In collaboration with Carl Rogers, a pioneer in person-centred psychotherapy, Gendlin developed a process-oriented experiential method, 'Focusing', for accomplishing the 'inner act' of making contact with 'felt sense' or internal awareness.[59] This structured attention to implicit or intricate knowing is in widespread use in Western psychotherapeutic practices. But it is designed also as a means of self-healing, providing 'a tool for people from all social strata and intellectual backgrounds to articulate their experiences' such that the capacity to 'develop new patterns of thought . . . is no longer limited to an intellectual elite, but is open to all'.[60] Gendlin's work has threefold value as a touchstone in the coming chapters. Firstly, his orientation towards personal therapy enables a seamless redirection of his influence on reading research towards the therapeutic impact of literature on the reader. Secondly, his emphasis on Focusing as a practice for everyone resembles The Reader's project in seeking to make great literature available for everyone who needs it, wherever they are.[61] Finally, Gendlin's insistence on the need to find and articulate the meaning of experience shares a clear affinity with the other therapeutic inspiration for this book, Wilfred Bion. The person who cannot find or is out of 'direct touch' with their 'inward datum' is 'lost', says Gendlin. 'Nothing is so debilitating as a clouded, narrowed or distant functioning of our own personally important experiencing.'[62] This book will return repeatedly to this guiding idea in the coming chapters.

6

Memory, time and loss: Encountering the past

The finding from our study that more intensely negative emotion was experienced in Shared Reading than in formal therapy can be in part explained by the fact that fiction and poetry were frequently a stimulus to forgotten or buried (emotional) pain. This phenomenon was so ubiquitous a feature of the reading sessions that the three mini case studies which follow are an initial snapshot only of a triggering of personal memory that we will see time and again across the reading instances that follow. But they magnify a process which (these instances collectively suggest) is going on more or less *implicitly* in literary reading much of the time and is thus potentially central to understanding why something so apparently soft as a story or a poem can affect something so intractable as physical pain.

Fay

During the reading of 'Mrs Manstey's View', Fay had been reminded intermittently of her own elderly and widowed mother, to whom she lived close by and whom she visited daily. On Mrs Manstey's indifference to sociability, for example, at the opening of the story, Fay had said she understood because her mother had not been out of the house for several years and had become accustomed to it. *People knock to ask 'how are you' and she just says 'I'm fine'. She doesn't want all that. She says half the time they're just looking for somewhere to go and yap. They're not interested in you.* Later, Fay recognized Mrs Manstey's daily routines and observances *through the way my mum has her own set little thing; she can't go out but she's got her garden and enjoys tending it.* Fay also spoke of the *frustration* she sometimes felt: *My mum's* *only got me. I'm an only child. I see her standing on a little ladder and I'm terrified she'll hurt herself. 'My legs are all right. While I can do it, let me do it.'* When she says that, I think I've got to stop assuming my mum's not strong enough.*

At the close of the session, which, as we've seen, moved Fay especially (*Her world is still there . . . that's lovely*), Fay became involuntarily very tearful. *Sorry. It's brought a lot of things to my head.* Viewing the video-recording of this moment later at the individual interview in which all participants in the study took part (see Chapter 5), she said: *I don't know why it did that to me. It just brought everything forward and I cried. To be honest I cried my eyes out when I went home. I was very down.* (This was verified by the words Fay used to describe her mood immediately after the session: 'Emotional; very upset'.) Fay went on to talk about how being sensitized to Mrs Manstey and what made her happy – *that it might be different to what other people think is happiness* – had *hurt* her by making her more aware of her inkling that she might be wrong in assuming *she knew what was best for my mum. It makes you think about the little things that are important and it's hard to – it's tuning in to what matters to people.*

The group leader, when interviewed, connected and contrasted Fay's response to 'Mrs Manstey's View', to her upset in relation to a story the group had read two or three months before. This was Elizabeth Bowen's 'The Visitor', in which a young boy tries to know, before anyone can tell him, the news he awaits of his mother's death. 'I can't let them tell me. It would be as though they saw me see her being killed!'[1] Fay picked up on this unusual formulation. *He wants to be alone where no one can see him because he doesn't know how he has to act, how people expect to see him, what the expression should be like on his face, in case it's the wrong thing. It reminds me,* she went on, *of when my dad passed away:*

> *We picked my son up from school. I remember it was a lovely summer's day, and we were waiting for the bus. And in the end, I just had to tell him at the bus stop. I remember he turned away and he took a few steps away from me, oh and my heart was, just for those couple of seconds. Yes, it was a horrible feeling. There wasn't a word out of him. And as soon as we got in the house, he went right over to my mum, buried his head in her shoulder and cried his eyes out. Oh it was horrible. God it was horrible.*

The turning away had to do, Fay reasoned, with her son's *first wave of shock. But I felt it like it was a reaction to me, because I had given him bad news.*

As the session ended, Fay said, *I can honestly say that's the only story I haven't enjoyed.* On Fay's PANAS for the session, negative emotions scored unusually highly. The group leader related at interview how she had worried at the time about the effect of this story on Fay to the extent that she hesitated over the choice of some texts thereafter for fear of producing further upset. However, Fay's response to 'Mrs Manstey's View' some weeks later – another *very real moment*, as the group leader saw it, where she experienced *a kind of sudden flash of understanding* in relation to her mother – made the group leader look differently upon the earlier session (Fay's memory of her own son in response to the young boy's situation in 'The Visitor').

> *It felt as though she had got in touch with something extremely uncomfortable to her, something she felt deeply guilty about and almost didn't understand herself. Because what happened was completely opposite to the intention she'd had. She probably felt it was deeply irresponsible, knowing Fay and how caring she is. And that picture which had stayed with her of her son turning to one side, and the pain she was giving him, was wrapped up with the loss of her father. She was the adult. But at that moment she was the child who had lost her father. She was almost confiding in her son, and that is a complicated knot of emotions. To find herself taken back to that place, it felt just so real for her; she was really right back in it and she didn't want to be in it. I think there was a sort of horror of – I suspect it is probably something she has avoided – but it just ambushed her.*

Where the model of 'Mrs Manstey', though saddening to Fay, seemed, as the group leader put it, *like a piece of wisdom she could take away which might help her with her mum in the future*, Fay's reaction to 'The Visitor' was by contrast *deeply disturbing and out of her control*. This intuition was vindicated by what transpired at the interview with Fay. While she remembered very well how 'Mrs Manstey's View' had *touched* her, she had no memory of 'The Visitor' or her own response to it, even with the video footage of the session there to remind her. It is as though the buried personal matter was simply *re-buried*, or 'avoided', once again.

*

There is a substantial body of literature in psychology indicating that disturbance or dysfunction in the retrieval of autobiographical memory (defined as 'the recollection of personally experienced past events'[2]) contributes to the onset and development of affective disorders – depression, most especially (closely associated, of course, with chronic pain). People with depression 'remember their past differently'[3] and their memories 'differ in form as well as in content'.[4] The recall of *overgeneral* autobiographical memory is a consistent characteristic of people diagnosed with depression. When recalling their autobiographical past, depressed people tend to summarize categories of events or recall ones that are repeated (occurring more than one time) or extended (lasting more than one day) rather than remembering a single or specific episode. Specific memories are ones that can be localized in time and space and contain the 'more concrete sensory–perceptual aspects of unique events, often including visual imagery rather than abstract, conceptual, verbal summaries of past experience'.[5]

Theoretical explanations for the occurrence of this phenomenon in depressed people tend to concur that avoidance mechanisms are at work. Episodic memories are experience-near: they are 'not only spatiotemporally unique but are also accompanied by subjective phenomenological details [sensory, affective, contextual]'.[6] When the memory is of past trauma or adversity, retrieval 'stops short', 'aborts the search for a specific event', in order to pre-empt the 'large and catastrophic increases in mood disturbance' that might be produced by affective content encoded in the fragment. 'The possible payoff for people with a less specific retrieval style [is that] they are less emotionally aroused by a negative personal experience.' While this 'dysfacilitation [of a cognitive process] might remain a flexible and helpful strategy in warding off negative emotions', such affect regulation comes at a long-term cost, partly because (as with avoidant behaviours in general) it can develop into a habitual and inflexible response pattern; but chiefly because autobiographical memory is 'central to human functioning'. Episodic memory is critical to the 'self-memory system', storing personal beliefs and values, developing 'an integrated and meaningful representation of one's self and one's life story'[7] and deeply implicated in the self's capacity to relive, reflect and introspect on one's subjective experience through time.

Chronic pain arguably creates its own predisposition to disturbances of autobiographical memory. In *Good Days, Bad Days: The Self and Chronic Illness in Time*, Kathy Charmaz gathers powerful testimonies of how chronically ill people, sometimes determinedly, often of necessity, live in the present. At one level, this is a survival strategy, 'a way of managing self while facing uncertainty': 'Living one day at a time mutes "negative" emotion – fear, guilt, anger, self-pity – [and] quiets feelings of being overwhelmed. . . . It allows people to focus on illness, treatment, and regimen without being overcome by dashed hopes and unmet expectations.'[8] At another level, living in the present is the ineluctable condition of chronic illness – 'the endless stretch forward of it', as Polly Atkin puts it in her autobiographical memoir, *Some of Us Just Fall*: 'day after day to get through, one after another. . . . Chronicity is [tedious] repetition – the repetitiveness and boredom of waking up each day feeling as bad or worse than the day before. The body's complaints vary but it always has complaints. In its difference, it is the same'.[9] What is a day like, asks Charmaz, for people living in this way? 'During a "good" day, they fill time. During a "bad" day they experience chaos. Filling time seldom involves structured activity. It means struggling

to rest, worrying . . . sometimes feeling barely alive . . . living on the edge –
the edge of control, the edge of coping, the edge of desperation.' Living one
day at a time, 'tacitly acknowledges . . . fragility'. The future is in abeyance,
unsettled or uncertain; the present expands ('time moves slowly and seems
empty') and also narrows ('choices dwindle, sorrow increases'); the past is
untrustworthy. 'During continued crisis . . . illness shoots by like a train that
has left the passenger behind, running after the caboose. Here the markers
of chronology [hospitalisation, treatment regimes] pile upon one another
in such swift succession that they blur together.' The past that has been
thus missed in the making becomes 'elusive' in retrospect, because 'losing
one's health can occur slowly [and] markers emerge . . . only when the
person becomes aware of lost function'. The past is not so much avoided,
then, as hardly there, barely available. At the same time, the past is often
all there is as 'a container for situating the self'. In chronic illness, often
enduring confinement, medication side effects, loneliness, exhaustion,
as well as poverty and confinement, people 'seldom have opportunities
or encouragement to change'. They 'lose a sense of evolving' when 'the
present offers scant material for constructing a valued self'.

> When the present marks a radical change, the past supplies more than the
> security of familiarity, it offers a foundation for reconstructing an altered if
> diminished self-concept [by] help[ing] one adapt to the present and shape
> a future. Taking strength from the past assuages fear.

When 'memory alone becomes the ultimate validation of self', a memory that
is unreliable leaves the self 'fragile and tentative'.[10]

* * *

Later in the interview, Fay was reminded by the video-recording of another
powerful and singular memory that had been triggered earlier in the session
on 'The Visitor', when the story was focused on the boy's perception of his
father's anxiety: 'Father didn't go to work now but walked about the house
and garden, his pink face horribly crinkled up and foolish looking, lighting
cigarettes and throwing them away again.'[11] Fay had said in the session:

> *The expression on his dad's face – he's not used to seeing that. I remember*
> *being scared when I saw my mum cry. She was always a happy person and*
> *usually when I came in she asked, 'What have you been doing in school?*
> *where have you been playing?' And just to see her – change like that. I*
> *didn't know what to do. My mum was crying. I'd never ever seen that on*
> *my mum before. She tried to hide it but it frightened me. I sort of backed*
> *away and she was saying come here. Then she had to tell me my grandad*

had died. I think as much as I loved my grandad, I was more upset about my mum being upset. It was just these tears. It was something I will never forget, never will. It stays with you.

More upset about my mum being upset is the syntax (compare 'It would be *as though they saw me see* her being killed!') of Fay's complexly 'knotty' family emotion. It reminds that behind the adult's saying, *I mean my mum's only got me. I'm an only child*, there is still the young girl's feeling, *I'm an only child. I've only got my mum.* This memory recalled what had at first struck Fay about the little boy in 'The Visitor' not wanting to hear from another the news that his mother was dead:

Oh, to run, to run quickly to somebody who would not know, who would think his mother was still alive, who need never know she was not! . . . He thrust his fingers into his ears 'I *know* I *know*!' he screamed. 'Go away, I can't bear it. I know I tell you.'[12]

He wants to know it already so he doesn't have to feel it, Fay remarked. *It's being scared of the emotion in a way.* Fay's implicit realization of the emotional logic of her own son's, and of her own child self's, reaction to loss and grief – (*He turned away, I sort of backed away*) out of sheer fear of feeling (*it frightened me, it's being scared*) – is inseparable from the story taking her *back to that place, right back in* the feeling. Expressive enactment, say Kuiken et al., is a form of enactive reading that – 'partly through the voice of the author and partly through the voice of the reader'[13] – 'implicitly blends the fictional world with what readers know, believe, or feel about their own lives'.[14] It differs from 'active self-projection into simulated situations decoupled from the here and now' (as proposed by Oatley et al.). Rather, the *felt meaning* elicited by the implicit blending of personal memory and fictional story, or of self and character, is 'more fully embodied and intimately present', engaging a 'reflective readiness', a kind of 'listening [for] affective resonance'[15] in the words of the text. *It's strange*, Fay said. *It took something like that – the story – to bring that memory out of me. To let that emotion out – it brings something on.* Thereafter, the group leader noted, there was a significant increase in Fay's engagement with the group and emotional involvement with the literature: *the release of the 'bad stuff' felt like a breakthrough, breaking the ice.* On re-opening and re-examining an earlier time, 'anchors to the past loosen and new possibilities for the present and future arise'. '[Re]appraisal of the significant event can itself become another significant event.'[16]

David

On this occasion, the group was reading Tobias Wolff's story 'The Liar' in which an adolescent boy is compulsively telling falsehoods about the dangerous state of his widowed mother's health. Initially, the talk centred around the possibility that the boy is seeking attention or feeling insecure, and the impact on the mother-son relationship. Susan suggests it *must be hard for the mum that the lies are about her*, because *it's not just like an embellishment; they're life threatening things he makes up, she coughs up blood, she's had leukaemia . . . You'd feel like he was wishing you ill harm.* David agrees: *There's a target to the lying isn't there? The mum is the target.* At length, Eve ventures: *Is this his way of coping with the death of his father?* Susan, too, wonders whether this behaviour is connected with unresolved grief around his father's passing, but is unsure why the boy *is picking on the mother, inventing problems about her.* Then David joins the conversation again:

> *Is he worried about the mother dying? 'cause dad's gone, mum could go. Kind of almost anticipating it in some way. My father died when I was eight. I remember worrying about my mum, was there something going to happen? I used to do things to protect her.*

Deborah, too, recognizes the anticipatory anxiety David attributes to the boy:

> *Deborah: I can remember when my mum died. I mean I was twenty-three, I wasn't a child but . . .*
> *David [interjecting]: It's still an early age though isn't it?*
> *Deborah: . . . and my dad had a heart by-pass operation soon after my mum died. I could see myself at my dad's funeral, after having just been to my mum's funeral. So in my mind – I wasn't telling anybody – but in my mind, I was going through those thought processes, like the boy's imagining. There wasn't anything 'wrong' with me. I was grieving. I was worrying.*
> *Susan: So, do you think he's trying to draw attention to – so people know his situation, maybe the way he feels or something?*

The group thought together about how this might be different to the attention-seeking that was discussed at the outset.

David did not speak again until a passage in the story where the boy-narrator recounts how his father, ill with cancer, had died while he was reading to him. 'I was alone in the house and didn't know what to do. His body did not frighten me but immediately and sharply I missed my father.' As it 'seemed wrong to leave him sitting up', the narrator continues, and as it was too hard to carry his father to his bedroom alone, he calls a friend to help him. When his mother returns, running upstairs calling her husband's name, and saying '"Thank God . . . at least he died in bed"', the narrator adds: 'This seemed important to her and I didn't tell her otherwise.'[17]

> *David: The lying started from there. He's telling lies for a reason. I have sympathy with him. He was young when his father died, and I know from my own experience, it leaves a massive imprint on your life. And even to this day, I've done things because of what happened in childhood. Nothing wrong, nothing bad or terrible but . . . I remember when my father died, for thirty years, if I passed an undertaker, I looked away, so I couldn't see it. 'Cause I was protecting my mother.*

Later, at the interview, David connected this experience to his diagnosis in adulthood with mild Obsessive Compulsive Disorder (OCD). Like the boy in the story, whose siblings had long left home, *it was just my mother and me*, he explains:

> *I didn't have any brothers or sisters. When my father has gone, I don't want my mother to go and I used to do things . . . because if I didn't turn off a tap or the oven, if I didn't do it three times something may happen to her. When you are a youngster, when you are on your own and you have got no, no siblings to talk to, your thoughts just retain there. I do feel that in the story.*

The striking shift to the present tense 'I don't want my mother to go' is like a direct confirmation of David's explanation of the origin of his OCD in arrested childhood emotional panic: *For thirty years . . . I looked away . . . I was protecting my mother.* David went on to connect the story to his son's OCD, which, he said, *really kicked in when my mother died – he was very close to her.* The relatively sudden onset of OCD symptoms in both father and son strongly resembles, significantly, David's description of the start of his current chronic condition:

> *One night I just went to bed, fine; the next night I went to bed and, oh, what is this feeling in my feet? It was more like sensations to start with, oh, can't sleep, got a sensation, and it gradually got worse, spreading to my hands. Strange isn't it?*

Moreover, when David described how the uncomfortable sensations in his feet and hands severely affected his sleep (he routinely managed an hour or two only), the behaviours of the adult in pain (*Sometimes I would be up most of the night, walking up and down in pain*) seems closely related to the repetitive habits of David as a bereaved only child (*your thoughts just retain there*).

***

Your thoughts retain there. This is a (profoundly apt) description of *rumination*, defined in clinical psychology as repetitive thinking: obsessively going over and over the same content, whether related to past events or current stressful circumstances, in a way which disables alternative problem-solving strategies. It is a key cognitive element of emotional disorders and predicts the onset and duration of depressive episodes.[18] It is also strongly associated with chronic pain, occurring frequently and in reciprocal relationship with not only pain, but negative emotions and sleeplessness.[19] Significantly, rumination is also implicated in overgeneralized autobiographical memory. In cases where negative self-representations are already in a state of heightened accessibility, the memory becomes 'captured'[20] or locked by self-related conceptual knowledge which prevents retrieval of the kind of sensory-perceptual detail associated with episodic memory. The more the mind short-circuits in this way, the more remote episodic memory becomes.

Charmaz describes this process in terms of the chronically ill person's changed relation to time and sometimes unregenerative relation to the past:

> Loss, unchanging time, social isolation [and] immersion in illness routines can foster situating oneself in the past, because the present may lack a sense of being really lived. In this situation, it is almost as if people observe rather than live their own lives. Although they do so in often invisible or implicit ways, people identify with some periods of time, events and experiences, but not with others. And their ways of viewing and relating to [past] time affect their emerging selves.

A common scenario is that emotions 'belonging' to a lost marker of the past – bewilderment, humiliation, shame, betrayal or loss – reverberate into the present. When they touch a 'shaky self-concept', bereft of definition and a sense of worth, they subtly 'shade', or merge with, and thereby demean it. A past only half-remembered can be invisibly *more* emotionally powerful than a specific memory, hiddenly working to create a diminished self in the present. Past emotions that are not redefined or 'transformed' 'etch deeper into the structure of the self'.[21]

***

The costs of David's condition have been severe, forcing him to retire early from a government post and, despite feeling himself to be a strong person and able to cope with life's difficulties, often feeling isolated from his family and depressed. Of his pain, David said:

> *It is coming from somewhere and they don't know where from, but it is primarily at night, as soon as I start relaxing, it starts.*

It is hard not to wonder whether chronic pain is the price David has to pay for any 'relaxation' of the vigilance (*If I didn't do it, something may happen to her*) involuntarily summoned in childhood by the experience of loss. The vigilance of rumination then recreates in turn the depression and pain. Notably, David said at interview that one way in which the reading group had helped him was in getting through bad nights. *I used to be crying at night sometimes, but now I can use the time better – to read instead.* Reading, one might say, now 'captures' David's thinking, 'retaining' his thoughts outside the cycle of OCD behaviours and rituals.

*

Innovative interventions for depression have recently been developed targeting disturbances in autobiographical memory. For example, Memory Specificity Training, in which participants repetitively practise the recall of specific memories elicited by positive, neutral and negative cue words, and Method-of-loci, an ancient mnemonic method that transforms items into visual images linked to specific locations, have shown amelioration in memory performance and several cognitive processes, including avoidance and problem-solving skills in people with depression. It is supposed that these results rest on memory 'reconsolidation',[22] the process by which experience is transformed into long-term memory. Reconsolidation occurs when an old memory is reactivated and updated with the incorporation of more specific material. In therapeutic models of memory consolidation, emotional arousal and the integration of new emotional-cognitive experiences into the reactivated memory are crucial components. It is significant that Fay's and David's responses exactly correspond to this model process. The story catalyses the memory in all its specificity and affective resonance: out of the emotional arousal comes a distinct cognitive shift of recognition: *It's being scared of the emotion in a way; when you're on your own, your thoughts just retain there.* Moreover, the fact that the memory is spontaneous and unforced suggests that literary reading might be a more efficient stimulus than programmatic memory 'training': 'Direct [spontaneous] retrieval is more rapid and less resource demanding than generative [cued] retrieval. . . . Memories recollected as a consequence of direct or "involuntary" retrieval tend to be more specific and less rehearsed than memories that are deliberately recollected in response to cue words.'[23] Memory recovered in this way, as we have seen, can 'flood consciousness [and] allow people to discover nuances within the event, to draw them out, and to scrutinise them . . . to receive another "take" on [an event's] meaning . . . that long remained unresolved'.[24]

The value of literary reading in relation to memory loss in particular may be a singular one. Recognizing that the affective resonance of a text is indeed at once less voluntary and 'more fundamental'[25] than conventional cognitive responses, moving certain readers at certain times according to its power to evoke personal memory and emotion, Sikora, Kuiken and Miall hypothesized that such effects were likely to occur with greater regularity in readers psychologically predisposed by experiences of loss, death and bereavement. Their rationale was founded on a property unique to literary discourse:

> On the one hand, stylistic features have the capacity to actualize their referents, to bring them to full and replete presence. On the other hand, stylistic features have the capacity to defamiliarize their referents, to make their taken-for-granted presence seem freshly unsettled.

The authors' model for this literary giving and taking away is the death-in-life figure of Coleridge's Ancient Mariner, which 'aesthetic object itself is figured as an apparition . . . experienced as palpably present and yet ephemeral and fragile'. Might it be, then, the authors propose, 'that for some individuals, the mournful mood that follows an impactful loss conditions a sensitivity to and engagement with aspects of a literary text in which this poignant interplay of presence and absence is re-enacted?'[26] To translate this thinking into the terms of the stories and readers we have just witnessed. In both 'The Visitor' and 'The Liar', the protagonists and their bereaved situations are tangibly present to these readers; while the key referent of each protagonists' experience (the mother, the father) is absent, dying or dead (lost or 'sharply missed'), and, at the same time, abidingly present, the occasion of the story. The proposition is that Fay's and David's experience of loss sensitizes them as literary readers to the tension generated by powerfully imagined presences, which even thus are unstable and vulnerable to passing away or to being rendered strange, unhomely. The 'defamiliarizing force of irrevocable loss – [has] the capacity to accentuate the workings of [literary] form, uproot us from our superficial and pragmatic selves'.[27] Moreover, Fay and David were perhaps at an optimum stage in life to be affected by these literary texts. Kuiken, Miall and Sikora found that the penetration of literature into life was less likely to occur among people who were depressed because of a recent significant loss, the initial period of psychological numbness seeming to preclude tolerance of, or confrontation with, the kind of re-saturation in grief which we witnessed in

Fay. Rather, 'feeling resonance' and 'self-perceptual depth'[28] were associated with depression in relation to an unresolved sense of loss occurring several or more years before. The authors' contention is that deep affective reading is perhaps 'dependent on the opening – or closing – of experiential windows during such seemingly inevitable life crises'.[29] Those who suffer life-trouble, we might conclude from this, have most to gain from fiction and poetry because they are primed by their suffering to be its best readers.

Let me test this proposition in relation to a different kind of loss and a different reader.

Mary[30]

Mary was the oldest member of the group, a widowed grandmother, and by far the quietest and most passive. But she became particularly and unusually animated and felt the need to speak out in relation to Elizabeth Taylor's short story 'Flesh'.

A middle-aged married woman, Phyl, taking a Mediterranean holiday as part of her convalescence following an illness, has an affair with a widower, Stanley, who had cared for his wife during her 'long, long illness'. When they spend the night together in a shabby hotel, they recall their respective partners, with whom each had enjoyed a rather limited and unsatisfying existence. 'He thought disloyally of the dead – of how Ethel would have started to be depressed by it all, and he would have had hard work jollying her out of her mood'; while Phyl was 'wryly imagining Charlie's wrath, how he would have carried on – for only the best was good enough for him, as he never tired of saying'.[31]

The group members discuss the tone of the couple's separate yet connected thinking – *You've got a real sense of the past, of their other lives being there at the same time. Stanley feels disloyal, but it doesn't seem like guilt exactly.*

> *Mary: This is how it should have been with his wife maybe. With his wife always being ill, I don't think he's really enjoyed . . . I think this is one of the best – he's really enjoying this because he's never had it before. And she's so **with** him, this woman. I think he's realizing what might have been, what's he lost really, what he hasn't had.*

Watching this moment at interview, Mary said:

> *I think that is the most I have ever said in the reading group. Yes, I have never spoken as much as I did. That is how I know it must have really got to me, the story.*

She repeated the words she used at the time as if in emphatic affirmation of the personal significance to her of the story: *What might have been. Because his wife was so ill, what he is having with this woman, he didn't have. And it is really what might have happened.* Then, slipping seamlessly into the husband's thought of his wife, Mary said, *Could I have had that, with her? And now it is gone. I think he's trying to recapture that – I think he wanted what he's missed.* Mary inhabits the live presence of the story in the group, then, on brief re-acquaintance, re-enters its reality at the interview. She then recalled an episode from her own youth, when she had fallen in love with an older man, a sailor, who put an end to the relationship when he went away to sea. *Of course I was broken-hearted*, Mary said with uncharacteristic depth of feeling, *really, really devastated.* Later he was sorry, and tried again; but it was much too late, and Mary herself had moved on. *Yes, well that's what might have been with me. Had he not finished with me, would I have continued with that relationship? [thoughtfully] I don't know.*

This does not feel like an account of lost chances and bad timing merely, but the location of some secret depth inside Mary, partially retrieved if only for the moment. Speaking of herself at another age and stage of life brings out of her and recovers someone just as real as the elderly widowed grandmother who now speaks. *It's as though*, said the group leader, the *story touched a vital spring.* This is not merely a 'might-have-been', characterized by loss or 'crisis'. It is an 'is', an access of energy, impelled by the force of literature and memory together – less an uprooting from the superficial, than a recovery of a resonance always potentially there, and secret even from Mary herself.

* * *

Chronic illness, as Charmaz's seminal work shows, changes one's relationship with time, and one's experience of time is inextricably bound up with one's experience of self. As Atkin puts it: 'A chronic illness is an illness which belongs to time. But it doesn't just last a long time: it changes time, eats it. . . . Time as you knew it dissolves into chronic time, as life as you knew it dissolves into chronic life.'[32]

This is 'crip time'. The term first emerged out of its informal usage in disability communities 'as a wry reference to the disability-related events that always seem to start late or to the disabled people who never seem to arrive anywhere on time'. Crip time now encompasses not only the need for extra time because of slower movement or access issues or equipment malfunction over which one has no control; it includes the ways in which the foregrounded physical needs of those living with disability or chronic illness determine the shape of each day, the way 'the present moment must often be measured against the moment to come' (as in 'if I do *this* now, I will have no energy for *that* later'). For people with chronic pain, especially, it recognizes what Alison Kafer calls 'time of undiagnosis: the shuttling between specialists, the repeated refusal of care and services, the constant denial of one's experiences, the slow exacerbation of one's symptoms, the years without recognition or diagnosis, the waiting'. It is a 'different orientation' to one's body and to time.[33] *Crip time is broken time.* It requires us to break in our bodies and minds to new rhythms, new patterns of thinking and feeling and moving through the world. It forces us to take breaks, even when we don't want to, even when we want to keep going, to move ahead.'[34] But crip time is also a whole 'reimagining . . . of what can and should happen in time'. It is self-consciously distinct from and resistant to the time which, as we saw in Chapter 1, is inseparable from medical definitions and conceptions of chronicity. It 'challenges the normative modalities that define time, such as productivity, accomplishment, and efficiency' and urges us towards different ideals, 'how we might begin to read these practices of self-care . . . as refusing such regimes'. 'Rather than bend disabled bodies and minds to meet the clock, crip time bends the clock to meet disabled bodies and minds.'[35] To this degree it is freeing, emancipatory, as Ellen Samuels suggests.

> The medical language of illness tries to reimpose the linear, speaking in terms of the chronic, the progressive, and the terminal, of relapses and stages. But we who occupy the bodies of crip time know that we are never linear. . . . Disability and illness have the power to extract us from linear, progressive time with its normative life stages and cast us into a wormhole of backward and forward acceleration, jerky stops and starts, tedious intervals and abrupt endings.

'Crip time is time travel.'[36] So, at many levels, is literary reading. It is not merely that it is often 'set' in a different time, though that can be part of the imaginative 'backward and forward' movement, of course. As we shall see again and again in what follows, whether fictional narrative or lyric poetry is in focus, the reading of literature offers an alternative temporal reality, one that exists at odds with (yet alongside) clock time, and which rarely, if ever, obeys straightforward linearity.[37] This is one way in which chronically ill people might be primed to the possibilities opened by reading. Inhabiting chronicity's alternative temporal reality creates a benign susceptibility to the imagined time sequences of fiction or the atemporality of lyric poetry, which in turn can more readily 'tune in' to the inner time of the reader; touching off a past self (as with Mary) which has something richer to give to the present than mere repetition or attenuation, albeit something often deeply troubling.

Indeed, what is striking about all three reading instances I have studied in this chapter is the power of the literary text to find secret affective resonances. The stories disclose, in Fay's and David's responses, a species of emptiness (*horror, horrible, I looked away so I couldn't see*), associated with the most primary relationships (mothers and others), which are not 'there' or present and yet which are potentially always there, and which, as we saw in Part I, can be central to psychic explorations of chronic pain. Neither the texts, the group leader, nor the discussion were directly in search of this psychotherapeutic terrain. But it could not be avoided even so. On the contrary, Fay was 'ambushed' by it.

It is with this in mind that I turn, in the next chapter, to consider individual experiences of literary shared reading alongside a programme of formal therapy. This will inevitably also keep in view, in the coming chapter and throughout Part II, the relation of the concept and experience of 'broken' time to ideas and practices dedicated to reshaping time, self and story.

7

Changing the story

The title of this chapter reflects a key linguistic finding of our study that participants' discourse in both CBT and Shared Reading was strongly marked by a tendency to tell and exchange personal stories. For this reason, the case studies in this chapter, and indeed across this part of the book, might be understood to be fulfilling, in many ways, the aims of what has come to be known as 'narrative medicine' which has gained considerable currency as an approach and practice within Western and, increasingly, global clinical care in recent years. There are, broadly speaking, twin rationales for the role of story-telling in medicine.

First, is the value of narrative for the patient. Serious illness, says Arthur Frank (in a foundational text for the turn to narrative in medical care, *The Wounded Storyteller*), is a loss of the 'destination and map that had previously guided the ill person's life'. Ill people need to tell their stories, in order to 'construct new maps and new perceptions' of their relationships to the world. This is especially imperative given that the story of illness that 'trumps all others' is the medical narrative. 'The voices of the ill are easy to ignore, because these voices are often faltering in tone and mixed in message, particularly in their spoken form. . . . [They] bespeak conditions of embodiment that most of us would rather forget our own vulnerability to.' Personal story at once challenges the hegemony of biomedical interpretations of illness by giving voice to what the latter cannot capture, and enables empowering expression to ill people whose experience is silenced and occluded by official accounts.[1]

Second, is the usefulness to the practitioner. As Rita Charon, doctor and founder of narrative medicine, asserts, in care of the sick, 'a scientifically competent medicine alone is not enough': 'Doctors need the expertise to listen to their patients, to understand as best they can the ordeals of illness, to honour the meanings of their patients' narratives of illness, and to be moved by what they behold so that they can act on their patients' behalf.'[2] Such expertise are especially essential in pain care.

> A complaint of crushing, sub-sternal chest pain (suggesting coronary artery disease, a condition we know how to treat) will elicit far more interest than will a complaint of migratory, non-localised, fuzzily described total body pain. Doctors are trained to make decisions, and many of them are intolerant of ambiguity or uncertainty, [leading to a] premature jump to closure [and often] to a faulty conclusion.[3]

Charon and colleagues have developed training programmes in 'narrative competence'[4] for medical trainees, which use literature to encourage the holding in mind of multiple possible interpretations in order to expand the trainees' 'bandwidth' when meeting with patients. Close literary reading is a primer for close 'radical listening'[5] in relation to patient's efforts to put their suffering into words.

These two key tenets of narrative medicine – the (patient's) need to tell and the (carer's) need to listen – are abundantly in evidence in what follows. But the emphasis of this chapter and the next is on the power of literature to shift, challenge or indeed *find* personal narrative. While the emphasis is by no means inimical to the practice of narrative medicine as it continues to evolve, there are areas of both overlap and distinction between the practices which are mutually illuminating and to which I return, therefore, later in this chapter (and the next) with the benefit of several more specific reading instances for illustration.

It should be pointed out that the CBT programme in the present study was not designed to encourage personal story-telling (though it proved to do exactly that). Delivered by the pain medicine consultants themselves, it was adapted for the particular needs of chronic pain patients. This was group CBT, incorporating relaxation training, stress and behavioural management, and coping skills. The aim was chiefly to assist patients in trying to manage the factors which may influence or exacerbate chronic pain suffering. CBT, as we saw in Part I, rests on the premise that a person's thoughts determine his or her feelings and behaviour, and thus a sustained attempt to change and inhibit negative and unhelpful thought patterns is the key to overcoming psychological distress. For pain consultants, the value of the therapy is that it can help sufferers to assess the effect that pain is having on their lives, and encourage problem-solving to reduce the impact of the pain on daily living. As well as addressing and alleviating such common by-products of pain as low mood, anxiety and sleep disorders, the key practical utility of CBT was to aid people in breaking out of a cycle of negativity which may prolong or worsen their suffering. *What we explore in CBT classes is the idea of accepting that this is how you are now, without that acceptance meaning that it's beaten you. You can be accepting of the situation without being hopeless. . . . It's a fine line to tread. People can't really move on until they've accepted the chronicity because they will be searching for that magic bullet, that thing that will cure them.*

The three case studies which follow centre on Holly, John and June and their individual and particular experience of being involved in CBT group therapy followed by Shared Reading. Within each case study, key implications and theoretical concerns are brought into play almost exclusively through the lens of the clinical perspective provided by the pain consultants who delivered the CBT. But in the course of the chapter as a whole, I will continue to draw on recent research on the psychology of reading and its reciprocal value as set out in the introduction to Part II (Chapter 5). That is to say, these empirical data offer living illustrations of some of psychology's experimental findings, while the latter help to illuminate the significance of the data witnessed in this clinical context.

Holly

Holly was one of the younger members of the group. In the first session, she responded to the open invitation from the consultant to describe the impact of her condition on her life:

> *It's the inactivity. You just stay in one place. I don't see anybody, I don't go anywhere. Prior to this I ran my own business. I used to run concerts, and I was really good at it. It was my life. I loved it. Now I don't even go to concerts, let alone put them on. I don't do anything with music anymore. I can't even speak to people about it. I haven't done anything all weekend except sit in a chair.*

Holly's discourse throughout CBT was characterized by the same strong sense of stasis – physical, social, psychological – and of deep loss:

> *I'm defined now by my pain. I'm defined by my pain rather than me defining who I am through – my actions. I am not who I was before pain. I feel very alone. I feel very, very alone with it, in as much as [long pause] I can't even describe properly how it feels.*

The passivity and subjugation visited upon Holly by her pain was evident in her demeanour. Apart from gently shaking her head at each *I don't, I'm not,* she sat very still, shoulders slumped forward, hands folded in lap, her facial features immobile, only her eyes darting quickly from time to time from the consultant to the other participants. There was, though, in that emphatic expression, **my** *actions*, the sign of an emotional response to her situation in need of release.

For the consultants, one of the therapeutic functions of the version of CBT they deliver is providing the space for their patients to talk freely about their experience of chronic pain. They explain that: *people who come to CBT have a lot of negative preconceptions as a result of numerous unsatisfactory medical experiences with other doctors, with the system, and in Accident and Emergency where their needs are not understood. Often close ones and family members have become frustrated or irritated listening to complaints about something which seems not to be there and yet never goes away.*

> *For many pain sufferers, CBT is the first space they have had directly to confront and reflect upon the often dramatic changes pain has wrought in their lives. There's no-one with chronic pain who wasn't without it at some stage in their life. With all of them, there is sense of loss of the person they were before they had chronic pain. The loss happens very quickly and intensely. It's like a bereavement, particularly for people who have been active beforehand. When physical activity is no longer a part of their life, it leaves a huge void.*

While group CBT gives sufferers the opportunity and permission to express their sense of a diminished life and self, its key focus, as expressed by the consultants, is on encouraging shifts in perception in relation to a condition which cannot itself be changed or cured. *There is an end in sight for people who are terminally ill; there is no foreseeable end to the suffering of those living with chronic pain.* The consultants recognized that finding a capacity for such inward change was often itself a slow and emotionally painful process. CBT *barely scratches the surface*, they said. But it was a start.

Holly is a good initial test case for examining the relative therapeutic benefit of CBT and literary reading, because she was very positive about her CBT experience. At interview, she spoke of the relief which came from exchanging personal histories with others who were struggling not only with the same symptoms but with similar day-to-day pressures. *It's getting things off your chest. I've got an eight-year-old child. And my mum worries so much, that I don't tell her how I feel a lot of the time because I don't want her to worry even more. So I don't tell anybody anything.* Holly in fact derived tangible practical benefit from CBT: the opportunity to expand on aspects of her distress led to a radically changed treatment plan, including a switch to an alternative prescribed medication, which improved her symptoms. She also *got a lot out of the sessions*, as she put it, *from an educational point of view.* In particular, she said, *it was a really massive thing to realize that most of our pain is emotional.*

The transcript below is from a session in which this learning is self-evident. The consultant has been summing up, from the words written on the flip chart, the ways in which the group have been defining their pain.

'It hurts'; 'depresses you'; 'low mood'; 'lack of motivation'; 'affects your socialisation'; 'lose your self-esteem . . . confidence . . . identity'. There's only one thing there that's about the sensation, the actual physical feeling and the rest of it is a lot of stuff that comes along with it, like feeling tired, feeling down, feeling isolated. Are there other feelings to add here?

The group volunteered *frustration, anger, worry* (about *how long I'll be on the tablets*), and *scared* (in case of further degeneration of the condition). The consultant then talked about the *vicious circles of pain* that are created as when, for example, feelings of low self-worth increase social isolation and intensify focus on pain. In this context he introduces the idea of avoidance (a key psychological element of the pain cycle, as we saw in Part I).

Consultant: Another way that pain can affect your quality of life is if you avoid doing something because you're worried it's going to hurt you.
Holly: I avoid anything that would cause me to be in more pain. Things like housework, cooking a meal, very much take a back seat, because I know I'll suffer for it the next day. I don't go anywhere I have to walk for any length of time, because I know it can put me in bed for a week afterwards. I can see how that feeds into the low mood, which feeds into the frustration, and the anger and the fear. Because I feel I'm letting my child down. He'd love to go to the zoo, and I won't walk around a zoo.
Consultant: It sounds as though you're feeling guilty too.
Holly: There's a lot of guilt there as well, yes.

At interview, Holly spoke of how CBT had helped her to make these connections for the first time: *Your low mood and the pain hold hands with one another, they're interchangeable.* There was little sign from ensuing sessions, however, that such recognitions were translating, where Sarah was concerned, into the shift of perception the consultants were seeking, away from the default tone and demeanour with which she joined the group. At the next session, for example, the consultant asked *How do you feel about acceptance?*:

Holly: You mean accepting that this is how it is and I've got to live my life with it? I'm not anywhere near that, no. On a scale of 1–10 I'm probably at minus 10. I went into a shop today and saw the news

> *headline, and that filled me with so much horror, because it said 'cold*
> *snap on the way' and I just know that I'm going to be in agony.*
> *Consultant:Any other worries just now?*
> *Holly:That you're not going to get better. Like this forever.*
> *Consultant:Yes, there's the getting worse part of it as well.*

In the session which followed, Holly recurred (as we shall see further shortly) to aspects of her illness story which she had spoken of before:

> *I take more painkillers so as to be able to work. If I could switch it all off and not worry about having to get up and go to work that would be better. But financially it would be crippling. So I'm sort of semi-crippled one way or the other but at least we're living.*
>
> *Consultant: [concerned]: Crippled is a very strong word.*

The session of Shared Reading which contrasted most starkly with Holly's way of being in CBT occurred soon after she joined the group. The poem was Elizabeth Jennings's 'Resemblances'. Holly, leaning forward, listened within intense concentration to the initial reading of the poem, to participants' first responses and to the group leader's re-reading of the first stanza, which begins: 'Always I look for some reminding feature,/Compel a likeness where there is not one.'[6]

> *Holly: Are you looking for normality?*
> *Group Leader: Normality? So not wanting anything unusual?*
> *Holly:You just want something that's [pause] familiar [nodding firmly on finding the word].*
> *Group Leader: I see, yes [nods too].*
> *Holly: And by going for the familiar [pausing and pointing at the text], it's saying if you just go for the familiar [shrugs, left hand opens casually] what about the new and exciting [right hand gesticulates rapidly] – you miss a lot.*
> *Group Leader: So it's kind of like having something in your head that you're actually looking for. And you're going to try and find it – whether it's there or not.*
> *Holly:Yes. Compelling a likeness. It's like saying, that's like that [pointing], making it fit what's known already.*

Notably, the group leader has to backtrack a little here in order to stay with the force of the first two lines of the poem (on the compulsion to look for and find what is familiar), because Holly has mentally already leapt ahead, to process the most important part of the stanza – its final two lines: 'Yet likenesses so searched for will yield none;/One feature, yes, but never the whole face.'[7] The exercise of Holly's vital intelligence, fully alive here to a new and unfamiliar thought, is apparent in her whole demeanour, which contrasted strikingly with her habitual stance in CBT. Her facial expressions and tone are animated (she and the group leader exchange gentle smiles of agreement throughout this conversation). Where, in CBT, Holly was often visibly in pain, shifting the position of her body with effort from time to time for relief, here her bodily movements correspond with the alertness of her thinking: after the first time she speaks, she readjusts her posture to sit upright as if purposefully preparing for her second contribution. The process of Holly's thinking is also markedly distinct from her default mentality and syntax in CBT. In place of the characteristically negative formulations (*I don't, I haven't, I can't, I won't*), expressive of aspects of her life that were all too known and familiar and apparently resistant to change, her thought develops through questions and pauses in which she is demonstrably seeking a way to make explicit the meaning of the poem, even as she has intuitively grasped it at once. Holly, at this moment, is the whole opposite of the person in CBT who was *just going for the familiar, fitting what's already known* and is (to use lines from the close of the poem) 'moved/Beyond the likeness to look behind'[8] what is habitual or automatic in every sense. What impressed the consultants most about such moments (when they themselves viewed the video-recordings at interview) was the fact that reading was producing in participants the outcomes which CBT was seeking, but doing so in participants' own time, at a point of readiness for change. *Some of the things we're trying to achieve in CBT – things we plant the seed of there, come out in a different way, an emotionally realized way in Shared Reading. You might think it's lost because the CBT course is over, but Shared Reading can bring things back or make them more individually 'have-able'.* What had seemed merely redundant moments in CBT now seemed part of a process which had helped Holly to *start thinking of herself, opening her to a more receptive state within the reading group.*

It is possible to make a direct comparison of Holly's responses in CBT and Shared Reading in relation to the same life material. As indicated above, in CBT, Holly's accounts were often repetitive (a symptom perhaps of the overgeneral memory we encountered in the last chapter and a tendency to recall negative memories more than positive ones). They recurred, in broad terms, to the same troubled beginnings of her illness:

Holly: I came out of an extremely abusive relationship, and was free for the first time in eight years. I had two children, I'd walked out – well, escaped – and started again. And then over a very short period of time I've become trapped by something else. That to me feels extremely unfair, very very unfair. To go from that to this.

When the group was reading from John Steinbeck's *Of Mice and Men*, where George paints a picture to his friend Lenny of a place better than the one in which they are now living ('It's ten acres. . . . Got a little win'mill. Got a little shack . . . an' a chicken run. Got a kitchen, orchard, cherries, apples, peaches, 'cots, nuts . . . berries'[9]), Sarah recurred to this time in her life. Having 'escaped' with her children (under a police escort) –

> *We found a house and it was – in a couple of days we'll move in and*
>   *it will be ours, you can have your rooms how you want them, we'll*
>   *have our own little space, safe without – have dinner whenever we*
>   *want, go the cinema, you can have friends round. It was lovely. It was*
>   *my front door key, my front door, my house. Then literally, I got sick.*
>   *Straightaway.*
> *Eve: Do you think the upset of the break-up eventually kicked off what*
>   *was always there, laying dormant?*
> *June: Like the aftermath? – years of stress and anxiety.*
> *Holly: Yes – it was like, 'It was all over' and then –*
> *Eve: Your body kept strong while it needed to.*
> *Holly: Yes [nods affirmatively] until I had the key and shut the door behind.*

At the time, the consultant was struck by how Holly was sharing the same difficult things she had been troubled or hurt by in CBT, but doing so with a new energy under the fresh stimulus of the fictional story. Not only was Holly's own story fuller and more detailed, her tone was upbeat, and her stance open. *It doesn't seem to drag her down. She even recovers the feeling of the initial joy of release – it was lovely . . . my house.* Patients such as Holly, the consultants explain, *define themselves more by their pain and by what they can't do than by what they can do or what they have done. Successful therapy should ideally reverse that tendency.* Here, the 'therapy' is the power of the literary text (to use the terms of reading psychology) to 'defamiliarize-refamiliarize' Holly's memory of a life-changing, traumatic event, calling it into play mimetically and allowing it to 'evolve in new directions'. 'Remembered feeling . . . does not remain merely replicative. . . . Either the original feeling is modified, or limitations of the original feeling are shown in such a way that a fresh feeling is created in its place.'[10] It is noteworthy in this regard that the connection and timing of Holly's illness vis-à-vis her prior domestic situation had been made neither by herself nor by the therapist in CBT: for the reason, as one consultant put it, that he *would not have wanted to be intrusive or indelicate, 'putting words into Holly's mouth'.* Eve makes this link on Holly's behalf, as it were, not as a professional but as a fellow-sufferer, and as a fellow-reader, a response which Holly described at interview by that same word she used in relation to her memory of a fresh start – *lovely.*

Later in the same session, the group read Edwin Muir's poem, 'Dream and Thing', in which the thing once dreamt of 'has come about', and has never doubted 'That everything is much like everything,/And the deep family likeness will come out'.[11] *I see that 'family likeness',* said Holly, pointing at the poem, re-reading and thinking hard for a few seconds, *as the similarity between the dream and the reality. The dream was 'bold' and we thought when it arrived it would be amazing and change our lives for forever. But it was – what it was.* Sarah used the analogy of starting a new business with excitement and finding it *hard-going to make it work [grimaces]. But if you think at least we've given up our boring jobs, you can see you've achieved quite a lot even though you haven't got where you meant to get. Look at what's gone right, not what's gone wrong. And 'trust' [a key word from the poem] in that. I mean the reality could surpass the dream.* Or, as the poem puts it: 'You may bring/From the dull mass each separate splendour out.' The dream is inside the thing, Sarah is saying in tandem with these words, if only we would look. It's hard to believe this is the same person who judged her capacity for acceptance to be *minus 10 out of 10.*

****.**

The animation and dynamism which struck the consultants on witnessing their patients participating in Shared Reading were not unique to Holly. On the contrary, the statistical component of our study corroborated the impression that the literature was an enlivening stimulus for all group members. One clear finding was the experience of a much greater range of emotion (as recorded by the two self-selected words recorded on the PANAS forms) in Shared Reading as compared to CBT, and the use of a far more diverse vocabulary (both cognitive and affective) for expressing these feelings. Words used to describe responses to CBT tended strongly towards the cognitive: 'interesting' and 'informative' were frequently used, for example, with emotion words generally restricted to 'relaxing' (by far the most common word used across participants), 'good session', 'enjoyed'. In Shared Reading, words used indicated a greater depth or strength of feeling – 'engaging', 'inspired', 'exciting', 'uplifted', 'content', 'very enthusiastic', 'involved', 'love the group' – and quite often were related to the experience of pain: 'helped to take my mind off pain', 'distracting from problems', 'enjoyable and great distraction from pain', 'helped with pain and anxiety', 'support'. This effect seemed to be reflected in 'feeling' words which had a 'physical' emphasis – 'energized', 'refreshed', 'awake', 'active', 'feel motivated' – many of which were often themselves leavened by a language of cognition: 'intrigued', 'interested', 'attentive', 'concentration', 'thoughtful', 'reflective', 'alert', 'determined', 'focused', 'deep', 'understanding', 'thought-provoking', 'descriptive'.

In a pilot version of our study, we had ventured that the access of life and energy, in mind and body, elicited by literary reading was consistent with the concept of 'flow'[12] – an optimal psychological state occurring when a person is completely engaged in a valued and intrinsically rewarding activity. First identified by Mihaly Csikszentmihalyi, in relation to the creative work of visual artists, and thence applied to absorption in learning, work, and creative and recreational activities, flow describes a point at which a person is engaged in a clear task, with strong concentration and focused attention, and where the demands of the activity are balanced harmoniously with a person's capacity to meet their challenge. It is associated with a loss of inhibiting self-consciousness, a heightened awareness of present being and of a sense of release from the pressure of ongoing time. Although a widely recognized concept in the area of positive psychology and Occupational Therapy, 'flow' has been relatively overlooked in relation to chronic pain. Those few studies which exist indicate a trend towards lower pain intensity while in flow, as well as flow's capacity to enhance concentration, motivation, self-esteem and potency in ways which distract from or enable modulation of the pain experience.[13] They also point out the special importance of making available flow-inducing activities for people with chronic pain, given the occupational deprivation among this group and the paucity of 'flow' opportunities in daily life.[14] Our own conclusion that literary reading is such an activity has recently received support from scholars in reading psychology who found flow to be not only a key predictor of the pleasures of reading literary narratives, but a central mediator and catalyst of multi-dimensional reading experiences, characterized by a sense of being present in the story world, identifying with protagonists and displaying optimal cognitive engagement.[15] Significantly, Csikszentmihalyi himself states that the idea of flow – its 'latent organising principle' – is a concept of 'psychic energy, or attention' first posited by William James.

> From the moment we wake up to when we fall asleep, we constantly need to invest attention in the tasks of everyday life. . . . Any information that registers in consciousness and there triggers an experience – any sight, sound, idea, or emotion – only exists because some of our psychic energy causes them to exist. Out of the millions of bits of potential information present in the environment, attention selects an infinitesimal subset and assimilates it into consciousness, thus creating a distinct experience.

'Attention is required to *have* an experience.' 'It is not surprising', Csikszentmihalyi states, 'that William James wrote that our lives consist of those things that we have attended to'. This 'fundamental insight'[16] perhaps applies with special force to a life lived with chronic pain. What struck the pain consultants particularly about our findings in relation to Shared Reading were the occasions when patients' emotion words indicated strong engagement ('focused', 'happy', 'energetic', 'proud') even when their pain scores were significantly high (7 or 8 on a 0–10 scale), and above average for the study. In relation to a condition which cannot be completely cured, where pain levels, however fluctuating, will always be more or less severe, the capacity of fiction and poetry reading to redirect psychic energy is in itself potent. Moreover, literary reading (as we witness it in these case studies) constitutes a special kind of attention-allocation – not only in respect of what is imagined as well as what is real, what is inside as well as outside, but insofar as the data 'selected' by consciousness in the present imaginary encounter can help reconfigure already assimilated life experience.

John

John, a husband and father in middle age, stated with characteristic energy and alertness when he first joined the CBT group, *I engage my thoughts on finding solutions to things.* This *persona*, the consultants felt, was very important to John. He offers a notably different test case for studying the relation of CBT and Shared Reading as 'therapies' for pain because of his sheer will to learn and to help change things for himself for the better: *I'm looking for an alternative [to the drugs]. You come to groups like this as an alternative way of moving forward. That's my ultimate goal: all these drugs – you start to rattle. You start thinking, crikey, I'm just popping pills: I never took tablets before.*

John's experience of and response to CBT is best illustrated by the final session, in which the consultant demonstrated the importance of overcoming negative thoughts, especially when something triggers a flare-up of pain. Negative thoughts give you negative emotions, the consultant reiterated, and the pain gets worse again. There is nothing to be gained by instinctively fighting it. On the contrary, the adrenalin produced by the distress of resistance only recreates the pain – another of chronic pain's vicious circles. For the patient's own sake, therefore, blind resistance needs to be replaced by something closer to tolerant acknowledgement. The necessity of combating negative thoughts is where the aims of CBT and the needs of chronic pain sufferers directly coincide and where the rationale of CBT for chronic pain is most clear.

The group was introduced to a number of conscious techniques to help sustain them in *not giving in to the negs*. The consultant explained that some people made use of pre-prepared mantras for when they caught themselves thinking negative thoughts. *They say to themselves, 'Well, hang on, I've been here before. I've been through it. I've always managed to get through it eventually no matter what happens.' Some people cling on to that thought.* John was particularly responsive to the challenge of positive thinking:

> *It reminds me of being in the army, when you go into operational theatre. If you're going down a road and the bridge has been taken out, you were told to think the bridge was still there. Because if you knew the bridge was out you'd turn round and go home.*

Thinking positively was at once John's inclination and disposition and an approach he rigorously and determinedly implemented at the onset of his pain. In the first session, John had described how his pain started in his lower limbs, spreading to his arms and hands, with the result that he could no longer use a manual self-propelling wheelchair, and was now reliant on an electric one.

> *I try to do things. I got into a rut when I took each day as it came. Now I try to have as many good days as I possibly can. My way of doing it is to try to re-activate the nerve-endings. I go swimming to try to regenerate something.*

Through taking up regular swimming, John had lost ten stone in weight.

> *On the days when I've got excruciating pain, I really give it, pull down with my arms. It's quite euphoric when you get out. For the first hour after the swimming, I feel absolutely brilliant and then it just [gestures a downwards slope] during the day. I try to go every day, but for the past month, I just haven't had the get up and go.*

John recounted how other challenges to his *really giving it* came chiefly from his family.

> *I have a workshop at home where I kept a mini-lathe, hand tools, power tools. There's a padlock on there now. I can't get at it. Not only that, they've even sold all the tools in case I find the key. So that has been taken away from me.*

He felt acutely the lack of understanding from his loved ones: *I think people remember me for what I used to be able to do. I used to be a party animal and some people think 'oh isn't it a shame', you know.* John was explicitly appreciative of the way CBT gave him some reflective distance from his problem-solving 'persona'.

> *It's quite cool that someone is seeing you from the outside. Sometimes you just get that blinkered view. I was coping too well, shouldering a lot, trying to go into my pre-pain mode. At some stage something has got to snap. So I've learned to pace myself.*

John had recognized how overdoing positive thinking – *trying too hard*, as he put it, *to be what I used to be* – could create its own negative circle.

What was striking about John's experience in the reading group was how often his 'pre-pain mode' was recalled – specifically memories of work – in response to the stimulus of the literature. In relation to Edith Wharton's short story 'Mrs Manstey's View', John remembered an elderly woman living on her own with whom he used to lodge when he was a long-distance lorry driver. *She used to expect me and watch for my wagon. She always knew when I was late.* When a young couple moved in next door and built an extension, *she couldn't see any more so she didn't know when I was coming.* Significantly, this memory, John's first contribution of length in the group, is not only a specific episode of his own former life but a poignant tale of somebody else's (emotional) pain. At a different register, Lennie's dependency upon George in John Steinbeck's *Of Mice and Men* prompted thoughts of when John was driving lorries on the continent, and would see another driver stopped along the way.

> *I'd pull in, and say 'What's up?' and he said I knew you'd be coming through. And then he'd be following all the way. It turned out he used to get lost all the time, you see. So what I think of this [pointing to the page] is that the two of them are together because they've got security with each other: there's a bond. They latch onto each other.*

Later, Michael used John's story as a way of understanding George's relationship with Lennie: *You stopped for your friend at work: you were very protective towards him. You were like George – you knew what you were doing where your friend didn't.* There was a sense in this exchange not only of something of the camaraderie John and Michael had formerly experienced at work being recreated, but of its being reproduced in a way that was not conventionally 'masculine'. At interview, John said of this moment: *We [i.e. men] don't talk in those terms. Not generally anyway. No, it is more practical situations that we talk about. It is not usually about how we feel.*

John verified at interview that these stories were often remembered by him again for the first time since giving up work altogether. He himself was struck by how all his stories came from a time when he was fit and able to do things. He also relished the fact that the stories came unexpectedly: *With pain, you are anticipating all the time, you've always got to plan. You can't be spontaneous anymore, and I was always spontaneous.* It has been a frequent finding of studies of Shared Reading, in fact, that, by stimulating recovery of lost aspects of being, the reading matter helps in 'bridging the gap between a current unwell/"abnormal" self, and a past whole/healthy self, [enabling] integration of fragmented parts of the self into a functioning whole'.[17]

The session in which the group read 'Mrs Manstey's View' closed with a reading of Norman Nicholson's 'The Pot Geranium'. The poem first describes the view from a high window of a crimson kite suddenly riding the air 'like a flight of racing pigeons', straining on a leash held by 'unseen boys' beneath:

> I turn from my window
> (Letting the bobbins of autumn wind up the swallows)
> And lie on my bed.[18]

John has been showing signs of wanting to speak for a few moments, as if waiting for the right time.

That bit in brackets – [reads it aloud] – I think it's the wind swirling the leaves [arms mimic the movement] and the swallows are caught up in the leaves. I used to see that when I pulled into Gretna [Green] services – all the swallows. I used to sit for hours watching.

As the poem goes onto to describe how 'white walls/Wrap themselves around me/...Thighs and spine/Are clamped to the mattress and looping strings/Twine round my chest and hold me', the group members speak of being 'cocooned by pain', 'the freedom gone' ('wind and sun/Are mine no longer, nor have I kite to claim them'[19]). 'We've got that "But" though', says the group leader. John nods as the group leader reads on:

> But there on a shelf
> In the warm corner of my dormer window
> A pot geranium flies its bright balloon . . .
> Contains the pattern, the prod and pulse of life[20]

The joy of seeing the kite has been assimilated into the geranium. I like that, said John. He then offered (for the first time) to read the close of the poem:

> My ways are circumscribed, confined as a limpet
> To one small radius of rock; yet
> I eat the equator, breathe the sky[21]

Those two last lines take me back to when I came off the ferry at Dover. I used to love driving. I'd just do what I do in the wheelchair now: sheer relaxation, 'Look what I've got in front of me'. That's where I breathe the sky. For an instant, John's wheelchair is vitally and energizingly connected to his past, rather than being an exclusively visible sign of his disabled present: more it is, momentarily, a *means* to peace in his current life, not solely a disadvantage to be determinedly overcome or compensated for. These (albeit tiny) shifts, not only in customary attitude but in familiar use of language – 'I breathe the sky' – are involuntary happenings, occasioned neither by self-will on John's part (joy, sheer relaxation, love, emotionally replace assiduously positive thinking here) nor as the intended outcome of formal therapy. Witnessing this moment at interview, John said:

> *The poem is saying everything is there combined for life. The geranium starts off as a small thing and then its life goes on and on doesn't it? There are little moments like that where you are just quite subdued and then bing, it is like the light comes on. And you can feel that happening inside like a connection.*

These inner connections are perhaps vital to the potential power of reading for chronic pain. As the pain consultants explain to participants in the CBT course, outlining the neuropathology of their condition as we encountered it in Part One: *There are specialized cells in your body whose job it is to detect and transmit pain and nothing else. Usually pain is picked up by one of these receptors, and impulses are sent through the nervous system to the brain:*

> *What happens in people with chronic pain, however, is that other nerves are recruited into this 'pain' pathway which start to fire off messages to the brain when there is no physical stimulus or damage. When we look back through case notes for people who have been coming for a long time, we often see that we're treating a different area to the one we were concerned with originally, and that's because the pain wiring system has set itself up and the body's joined in with it. But the body can 'unjoin' again. Nerve blockers (drugs) are one way; reading might be another.*

The group leader observed of John's response to 'The Pot Geranium' that the way his very language came alive (*bing, the light comes on*) *is a kind of testimony that the inner connections which happen in reading can galvanise the over-rigidity of nervous impulses or 'pain pathways' by firing new messages or producing a mental 're-wiring' of kinds.*[22]

***

It is such recognition of the potential for literary works to rewire thinking which sets an activity like Shared Reading apart from the aims and practice of narrative medicine. In fact, the latter are arguably more fulfilled by the group CBT delivered by the pain consultants than by Shared Reading. In many ways, this is unsurprising, given that the consultants' relationship with their patients largely fits the prototype narrative practitioner suggested by Charon. The personal-biological dimensions of ill health become clear only through a knowledge which accrues through the doctors 'grow[ing] with' their patient and getting to know their lives. 'To understand what disease a patient might have requires schooled longitudinal curiosity about that person's state of health. Sicknesses declare themselves over time, not in one visit to the consultant.'[23] The sentiment is resoundingly echoed by (retired) British GP Iona Heath who says (in a volume dedicated to narrative-based medicine): 'Stories are told throughout medicine, but only general practice offers the possibility of doctors and patients sharing their stories over a lifetime.'[24] It is of immense significance therefore, that the pain consultants feel that *we're almost treated as a GP* insofar as *people present us with problems that aren't related to pain*, seeking what is essentially *day-to-day care*:

> *A lot of our patients say that the simple greeting 'How are you?' fills them with dread because they don't know what to say. They're worried that they will bore those who ask so they keep it to themselves. Being able to come to the clinic and to express how they're feeling is an important part of the therapeutic relationship. I think we fulfil that role more than GPs do now, the role has changed so much. A lot of medicine is protocol and algorithm driven, whereas, in the clinic, people are coming to see you because, with your experience and knowledge, you're not just following the protocol.*

Above all, they say, *we try to validate the pain. A lot of people have been told it's all in their head – we need to get that idea out of the way.*

As we have seen, though, the consultants were aware that the personal stories in CBT were often characterized by a language of lack. Even where stories were apparently being shared for the first time in the group, there was a sense that they were already rigidified in some way, in danger of confirming stasis rather than encouraging change or movement, and reinforcing perceptions of self which were already established or 'fixed'. This intuition was confirmed by the linguists on the study, who found not only that there was a strong emphasis on a sense of diminishment or subtraction, things 'taken away' by chronic pain: participants in fact focused exclusively on their pain with 'no thematic deviation'.[25] This is the danger of the illness narrative, of course, that (especially through public repetition or familiarity) it can become a default attitude which hides the suffering reality which it contains. This is especially true of chronic pain as Jean Jackson points out: 'Chronic pain as a topic for description and discussion . . . easily slips toward numbing boredom for the casual observer and often for the person experiencing it' because it 'achieves no transcendence'. 'Resistance to being transformed into something meaningful – from an unmediated evil to a mixed good – . . . threatens a collapse into a counter-narrative where nothing happens beyond the repetition of a meaningless and inarticulate suffering.'[26] This not only obstructs change but, as the narrative is granted 'obdurate qualities', can intensify the damage. Charmaz gives the example of how 'crushing moments' of remembered shame can be relived 'over and over and over'. 'Shame lasts . . . implies failure . . . strips away self-respect' and bespeaks and fosters 'a fundamental uncertainty about self-definition and self-worth'.[27]

The stories elicited in Shared Reading, by stark contrast, were often a form of restoration, via the new stimulus of the literary story or poem, of what participants still *did* have (memories, feelings, thoughts, experiences) rather than a rehearsal or repetition of what they had lost. This is an alternative model of 'recovery' – one more suited to the insusceptibility of chronic pain to simple 'cure' – which comprises rediscovery of old or forgotten, suppressed or inaccessible, modes of being as much as the discovery of new ones. It is the kind of reclamation, valuing and use of past self and time which, Charmaz found, lends 'strength' to the frail present of chronic illness, 'recombining and restructuring' past, present and projected future selves in 'different, shifting', rather than obstinate, ways.[28] Shared Reading, in short, helps recover, and promise, a whole person, not just an ill one. As one consultant put it, *When people are in CBT, they are people with pain. When they're in the reading group, they're people with lives.*

June

June's experience of the reading and CBT groups helps to point up some of the divergences between the two activities as identified by the consultants. June offers another perspective again, one very different to that of either Holly or John, because she was possibly more resistant to CBT than to pain itself. A mother of four children and a grandmother of five, June had been a nurse all her working life. She was now also carer for her ageing and unwell parents. Before her pain condition *stopped me from doing all kinds*, June had always been formidably active, involved in sundry community activities and, in addition to her nursing career, had trained and worked as a social worker and counsellor. One reason she gave for her *negative* experience of CBT was her occupational background. *The worst thing to be, right, is a – professional in a professional group? I've run groups in my previous life.* She was aware that she appraised the process too consciously and that this was an obstacle to her engagement: *I don't know whether I was ever fully involved in CBT.* She also had reservations about CBT's *professional* approach. *I understood what we were doing, why we were there. But it's like in some respect you're looking from a script. I felt as if we were just going through the motions somehow.* June spoke relatively rarely in the CBT group in fact. In the first session, like the other participants, she told something of the impact of pain on her life. *I can't multitask the way I used to. I can't concentrate. If I've got to plan anything I can't – it just sets my head off all wonky. My grandson says to me, I've got a spongy brain.* Occasionally she mentioned the pressures of work and family, her constant tiredness and the difficulty she had in meeting her own needs. *I can't be sick. My mum and dad can't see that I'm not well. It's not within the parameters of what they perceive me as.* (I am instinctively reminded of Jean Jackson's finding that carers were over-represented among chronic pain sufferers.) Once she spoke of the isolation and frustration she suffered as a result. *It makes you very lonely because nobody understands.* Mostly, however, June would speak simply to indicate agreement. When Holly – in response to the consultant's question *How do you feel about acceptance?* – declared *on a scale of 1–10 I'm probably at minus 10*, June simply said, *Me, too.* This defeatist tone and tendency within the CBT group was continuous with her summing up of the experience at interview afterwards. *I didn't get anything from it. Nothing has happened from it. I'm sorry I went.*

June made a stark comparison between her experience of CBT and her response to the reading group. *I've thrown myself into the reading group, quite, you know, what's the word, wholeheartedly, 100%. I threw myself into CBT about 10%.* This was corroborated both by the video footage June viewed at interview and her response to it. So, for example, when watching the group discussion of 'Mrs Manstey's View' she exclaimed: *Oh Mrs Manstey. Oh I loved Mrs Manstey. I loved her, I felt so sorry for her. It affected me so much. I cried when she died. I love her.* In the session itself, June (as the reader may recall) had connected the story to her father's loneliness: *This upsets me, you know, 'cause my dad can't, my dad doesn't go out. . . . Is that all there is for him? That he's content like that?* The concentrated and emphatic energy of tone, facial expression and physical stance with which she uttered, *This upsets me*, truly pained as she was at this moment, is virtually identical to the tonal register of body and voice in which she later recalled, at interview, how the story 'affected' her (*I cried when she died. I love her*). Both interviewer and June connected this coincidence of affect (underscored by June's instinctive use of the present tense) with the fact that June several times returned to thoughts of 'Mrs Manstey's View' in later reading sessions, as though story and character had involuntarily formed an emotional touchstone for her. *Every time something happens I say remember Mrs Manstey.* June noted with surprise that this reading session had recalled to her a CBT class in which *we had a significant discussion about how people were taking our choices away*; the recollection had arisen because the story had prompted June to recall her role as a counsellor in palliative care. She remembered the difficulty of *trying to explain to families that it's not really what they want that counts when a person is dying.* In the course of the Shared Reading session, therefore, June had been first a troubled daughter; then the counsellor who could understand the daughter's sorrow and help modify it; then the pain sufferer herself, able to reflect on the therapy she has received in relation to it. Where June's professional background had been one of the factors which blocked her personal involvement with CBT, here it returns freely, richly intermixed with her personal emotional and physical pain. This is what the pain consultants mean when they say that in Shared Reading people have lives. Pain is a part of their story, but not the whole of it.

June's attitude (bodily and mental) in CBT came as a shock to members of the research team who had seen June only in the reading group, where she was often the most vocal and thoughtful of the participants. Take, for example, her contribution when the group was reading Christina Rossetti's poem 'Shut Out'. In the early stanzas, the speaker looks between the iron bars of a closed barrier to 'My garden, mine, beneath the sky,/Pied with all flowers bedewed and green', and asks the spirit who keeps the gate, 'Let me have/Some buds to cheer my outcast state'. In response, the spirit ('Blank and unchanging like the grave') silently builds a wall leaving 'no loophole great or small/Through which my straining eyes might look'.[29] The group members talked of being *cut off from all the beautiful things that you can't have, can't get at. Like prison,* says one. *Like death,* says another.

> *June: The spirit builds up this wall so you can't even see what you've lost. You've got to say goodbye to the things you've had to leave behind. But if you have a dream or something you were looking forward to and then you had to let it go – would you rather have a little bit of it, be able to see what you've lost, or just put a wall up?*

June, as she often did, offered to re-read the final two stanzas.

> So now I sit here quite alone
> Blinded with tears; nor grieve for that,
> For nought is left worth looking at
> Since my delightful land is gone.

> A violet bed is budding near,
> Wherein a lark has made her nest:
> And good they are, but not the best;
> And dear they are, but not so dear.[30]

It's make do and mend, said one group member (Eve); *you can make something worthwhile out of whatever situation.* June wasn't so sure.

> *June: They've lost things, yet they've still got a violet bed, a lark. But that's not. . . . Maybe it's more a mix and match at the end there. [Using both hands, palms up, to balance each half line.] 'Good they are' [left hand up, right down], 'but not the best' [right hand up, left down], 'And dear they are' [reverse], 'but not so dear' [reverse]. I feel like it's giving with one hand and taking away with the other.*

Body and mind are working intensely together to tease out the delicate poise written into the repeated parallel structure of the final two lines, where twice over the second half line modifies, without wholly opposing or cancelling, the import of the first. Sally uses these technical resources of the poem to steer herself and the group away from an acceptance of loss which seems instinctively to strike her, when she herself is inclined that way, as too easy (*Yet they've still got . . . But that's not*). *Yet, but, maybe,* pauses and hesitation: this is the syntax of a mind in dialogue with itself about relative gains and losses and to what degree acceptance is achieved, or is even possible or appropriate. It is remote indeed from the person who *can't concentrate* and whose brain is described as *spongy*; it is also a subtler refusal of mere acceptance than Sally's readily acquiescent *Me too* in CBT. Where that was passively close to the CBT group's reactively negative *script*, the script of the poem, by contrast, provides a discipline more testing than that of professional therapy and a mentality in relation to 'lost things' that is not rehearsed, habitual or known.

* * *

One of the consultants at the pain clinic described Shared Reading as *a doorway to effect change in cognition*:

> *Ingrained patterns of thinking are common to everyone with chronic pain and have an adverse effect on quality of life. What we try to do in CBT is to get people to recognise that pattern of thinking and to rationalise it. Shared Reading can help with that process through the immersed exploration of the characters, through vicariously examining their behaviours and emotions, rather than it being personal straight away. And you can choose whether or not you wish to think about the emotions that those characters*

in the literature have evoked in you and why that might be. Unshakeable beliefs can be challenged directly but when it's removed from you as an individual – it's a character in a book – it's easier to change your mind or to take a different perspective. It's recognising self, sometimes in a good way and sometimes in a more challenging way.

While cognitive change is the goal, what *opens the door* to thought is emotion.

CBT is an intellectual understanding of concepts – we're tapping into one part of our patients' thinking but we're not tackling the emotional side of it. We know that pain is essentially an emotional thing. This is why it is important that Shared Reading is operating on a much more emotional level than CBT.

This intuitive summary of the process of literary reading as understood by the pain clinicians helps to show where and how the psychology of pain and the psychology of reading usefully meet. As we saw in Chapter 5, the notion that literature can de-automatize perception is central to psychological theories of reading. 'Foregrounding is the opposite of automatization . . . the more an act is automatized, the less it is consciously executed; the more it is foregrounded, the more completely conscious does it become.'[31] It is because the 'strikingness of literature occurs against a background of familiarity and habituation'[32] that it impels flexibility, reconsideration and reshaping of our perspectives. David Miall, one of the founders of the empirical study of literature as it has developed in the twenty-first century, regarded the mobilization of personal affect as a precondition of deautomatization. Opposing the 'impoverished' (and now outmoded) approach to narrative comprehension using information processing models, Miall insisted that *feeling* not cognition was the prime mover in response to narrative fiction, correctively situating affective response as central. 'The emotions invoked by narrative episodes and their outcome' – 'where the reader's own concerns and anticipations are implicated from the first paragraph' – enable the reader 'to rehearse the implications for the self of the situations and events portrayed on a symbolic stage . . . in isolation from the world of action'. In particular, it is 'in conditions of uncertainty, when narrative elements cannot readily be assigned to existing schemata' that the latter are most susceptible to redefinition, modification or suspension:

Reading a literary text is an interaction between an emotion-directed feed-forward mechanism that enables constructive responses to be made to forthcoming episodes, and a defamiliarizing mechanism that restructures the reader's anticipations and feeds back corrective information to the initiating emotion. One effect may be to alter the emotional valency of existing schemata, and thus their relationship to other elements within the cognitive system, as well as to bring into being new (and possibly more adaptive) schemata.[33]

We have seen this emotional-cognitive revaluation in both micro and macro operation in individual and collective responses to 'Mrs Manstey's View', in Mary's response to 'Flesh' and in David's to 'The Liar'. Narrative at such times is not simply a model or vehicle for expression of the personal, but an intervention *in* the personal, a recalibrating force. And this effect is by no means restricted to narrative, as we have just witnessed in the last case study, a crucial matter to which I return in the next chapter. I close here, however, with a brief vignette in relation to what might be regarded as the Ur-text in modern Western literature of a defamiliarized schemata, Charles Dickens's *A Christmas Carol*. In the session which concluded the group's reading of this novel (the first lengthy work of narrative fiction the group had encountered), they read together the final chapters of the story, in which the Ghost of Christmas Yet to Come grants Scrooge a vision of his own deathbed. 'He lay in the dark empty house, with not a man, a woman, or a child, to say that he was kind.'

> 'Spirit!' he cried, tight clutching at its robe, 'hear me! I am not the man I was. I will not be the man I must have been but for this intercourse. Why show me this, if I am past all hope! . . . Assure me that I yet may change these shadows you have shown me, by an altered life! . . . I will honour Christmas in my heart, and try to keep it all the year'.[34]

> *Eve: 'I am not the man I was.' It's the change of perception that's important. He's learned not just who he was but who he needs to be. Even the smallest things can teach you.*

The consultants were struck, on seeing this, by how the very premise on which their version of CBT is built – that the all-important change is one of perception – is not imposed upon participants but freely discovered by them personally. *They find what they need to know in their own way, as if it is coming from themselves individually not from outside.*

> *Eve: [pointing to the words as she reads] 'Assure me that I may yet change these shadows you have shown me by an altered life?' Isn't this sort of like someone writing a story, and reading over what they've put in the story and then – [energetically] they go back and – and alter it. The phantom is showing that the future can be changed if it wants to change. [quoting] 'I hope to live to be another man'.[35]*

And alter it is palpably a message new-fired, like a regenerated nerve impulse, set going by the text. Unlike CBT, Shared Reading creates change, and belief in change, precisely by not demanding it. The *story* achieves CBT's ambition of putting the same person in a different place, by modelling that change in Scrooge.

When the book was finished, the group broke into spontaneous applause, half for Scrooge's accomplishment (*it's a new experience, an exaltation, elation, like being given a second chance*), and half for their own. Either way, this was a wholehearted expression of joyful release. This is literature *doing* narrative medicine, excitedly, in action.

8

Finding a language

Where the chapters so far in this part of the book have been largely concerned with how literary reading can help *locate* or *change* aspects of a person's self and story, this chapter is more specifically concerned with the power of literary language not only to find but also to *express* pain and suffering.

This notion and claim is apparently at odds with much work in the field of pain. Since the publication in 1985 of Elaine Scarry's seminal *The Body in Pain*, it has become almost axiomatic to assume that language is inadequate to the purpose of such expression, and Scarry's thesis remains a critical yardstick because this assumption is cogently underwritten by chronic pain sufferers' lived experience. As John put it in a CBT session: *I always used to struggle when a doctor said 'Describe the pain' or 'Describe how you feel'. Describing it to myself, I struggle. I would say 'It kills me', but then you have to look for ways and means to tell other people – it just becomes a mish-mash.* And, as Holly's testimony witnesses, the issue is severely compounded by the power invested in the official (and severely limited) language of health and social care. *When I had an assessment [for disability benefit] in my home, the person just couldn't empathise. They have their own terminology: is this chronic illness or is this mental illness? – that's what they want to know. There are no grey areas. So they'll lump you into one or the other. And it's frustrating because you can't accurately describe what is wrong with you.* As we have seen, the pain consultants used CBT to encourage patients to identify their suffering as a way of helping them to think about their condition rather than being simply subject to it. The explicit naming of, for example, fear, guilt, avoidance, frustration, might be essential not only as a first step in recognition and acceptance but in externally framing and discriminating damaging inner emotions otherwise experienced amorphously as 'pain'. Nevertheless, the consultants were aware of the almost equal danger of thereby imposing a vocabulary and limiting the latter's potential range. These same nouns might become an automatic language that not only disauthenticates but helps to produce internal reality. As with the word 'pain' itself, when it becomes a settled part of one's mentality, definitive names can impoverish not only one's language but one's sense of oneself subjectively.

In her fascinating and often arrestingly beautiful *Perceptions of Pain*, Deborah Padfield has shown the formidable eloquence of visual images to communicate the feel of the body in pain. Padfield, an artist and chronic pain sufferer, collaborated with a pain consultant and his patients at the pain clinic at St Thomas's Hospital in London to explore and co-record their experiences of pain in photographic images which could be used in subsequent medical consultations. The challenge 'was not to make shareable the external ravages or indications of pain, but something of the internal invisible qualities inherent to individual pain', enabling pain patients to 'project the private sensations and experiences of pain – its associations, intensities, qualities and significance – outwards on to the publicly accessible surfaces of canvases and photographic plates'. Among these private experiences of pain, says Padfield, is the need to prove its very existence, as much to oneself as to a doubting world and medical establishment. 'If there is a moment when it does not appear to exist, then the horrible possibility is raised that it might never have existed at all! If the pain that was so debilitating was never real, what else in the world is also unreal?' The necessity of proving one's pain 'increases a person's experience of pain, trapping them within one of the few certainties left to them'. One key value of a photograph, therefore, is that the 'pain can be trapped within an external representation . . . instead of within the body' and 'once that photograph has been seen and accepted as "real" by others, the sufferer no longer has to prove the existence of the pain and the pain is reduced'. The production of 'a visual language for pain' was the outcome of weeks of collaboration during which an artist composed images of objects and ideas suggested by and directly worked on by the patients using experimental materials and techniques (cement and concrete; glass and water; fire and ice; and cutting, tearing, stitching and drawing). One series of images depicts first the disassembled internal mechanical parts of a clock and then their superimposition upon a human face. It is accompanied by this commentary from the patient (a former postal sorter on the night mail): 'Time-keeping was very much part of my life. It is in me here. . . . When I was injured, I couldn't move at all. I was wearing a watch, so I started taking apart all the tiny pieces and putting it back together again. . . . You can't dismantle the body like a clock.' The value of these images as a 'shared reference point'[1] for more equal and mutually beneficial dialogue between patient and doctor was demonstrated in a subsequent study which showed that 'the materiality of the images [brought] patients' experience directly into the consultation'. 'Affecting and visceral in their directness [they opened] up a different kind of space from the traditional verbal encounters with medical practitioners',[2] encouraging a more personal language, more emotional disclosure and an increase in the patient's proportionate contribution to the conversation. In thus strengthening the agency of patients within the unequal hierarchies of clinical medicine, by providing 'a bridge' between private suffering and medical understanding, it is above all the primacy of the visual medium in accessing what is lonely and isolated in the pain sufferer which chiefly motivates Padfield's work.

> Most of the sufferers I worked with describe the space they inhabit when the pain is severe in terms of blackness, emptiness and aloneness. It is reflected in the images produced, many of them portraying objects floating in, or isolated within, a black space. The associated feelings are frequently of fear and being out of control. . . . What is it that this darkness represents? It seems as though it takes us back to a primal space where words have not yet formed. . . . It requires a language which works on a more instinctual and primal level than words.[3]

In her influential 'provocation' regarding the limits of narrative as a tool in medicine and clinical practice, Angela Woods cites Padfield's work as offering a challenge to 'narrative medicine's foundational, normative claims that self-expression through narrative is fundamentally healthy and desirable, especially in the case of illness' and as an exemplary alternative to verbal and linear representation. In a climate in which, as we saw in the preceding chapter, narrative is increasingly regarded (across clinical, social science and humanities disciplines) as providing privileged access to the individual experience of illness and is offered as the principal means by which a person who is ill can express their sense of a changing self, there is often an assumption that 'a person's narrative [is] coextensive with their subjective experience, their psychological health and indeed their very humanity'. This has the potentially damaging effect, Woods argues, of promoting 'a specific model of the self – as an agentic, authentic, autonomous storyteller; as someone with unique insight into an essentially private and emotionally rich inner world; as someone who possesses a drive for story-telling, and whose stories reflect and (re)affirm a sense of enduring, individual identity'. Not only is the reification of a Western, middle-class, confessional model of shaping and expressing subjective experience potentially exclusive, argues Woods; it also precludes the possibility that illness might impel a present-focused orientation rather than an inclination towards narrative's temporal sequence and arc.

> Does illness propel us in the direction of diachronicity, forcing us to mourn a healthy past which cannot be recuperated and a future which feels more

fraught, more finite? Or is it the case that illness demands instead that we attend to the right now, either because pain returns us to the immediacy of the body, or because the uncertainty of the future encourages us to invest more intensely in the self-experience of the present?[4]

These rightly remain open questions. As we have seen in Chapters 6 and 7, chronic illness in particular reframes the self's relationship to time, and which time frame takes priority, in terms of locating self-concept and self-definition, changes 'kaleidoscopically'. 'Ill people's self-concepts may shift their locations in the past, present or future at different points in their illnesses' so that 'a person who has been tied to the past or future may come to live in the present and to see self as situated within it'.[5]

Recently, Sara Wasson has brought both the example of Padfield's practice and the implications of Woods's polemic directly to bear on chronic pain in her critical-creative writing project, 'Translating Chronic Pain'. Wasson's premise is that chronic pain's 'invisibility', not only to health practitioners but to friends, family and the general public, is in part owing to the fact that 'chronic pain can be hard to turn into story, thanks to its jagged unpredictability, and its resistance to clear causality and cure'. Chronic pain does not lend itself either (as we saw Jean Jackson also contend in the previous chapter) to established forms of illness narrative, the sickness memoir or survivorship story, wherein resolution or restitution is achieved. The aim of Wasson's project is to 'better represent chronic pain experience by disrupting existing expectations of illness memoir' and inviting instead '"flash" illness writing: fragmentary, episode-focused, short-format work, both word and image' expressing the experience of pain in 'glimpses' or 'moments'.[6] The project has collected into an online anthology one hundred such prose and poetry fragments whose brevity and public availability are intended, as with Padfield's images, to stimulate the use of the material by healthcare practitioners and medical educators to enrich the perception and understanding of the suffering of people living with chronic pain.

The anti-narrative emphases of these projects and polemics resonate with the definition of 'crip time' introduced at the close of Chapter 6, which, Kafer says, 'exists in stark contrast to "curative time"',[7] the temporality of the ableist orientation towards inevitable (and in the case of chronic pain, mostly futile) medical intervention in the service of an illness-to-health narrative trajectory. Yet in thus resisting the tendencies and trajectory of the developmental narrative arc, it is possible that these challenges to linear, sequential conceptions of chronic illness take too little account of, for example, what living in the present can feel like – what, as an ontological experience, it is – as we encountered it also in Chapter 6. 'A chronic illness is the end of time', says Atkin. 'It is carrying on. It is enduring. It is unendurable.' 'This is time snapped into fragments, into disconnected phrases. . . . Time becomes an endless, looping condition experienced through the body. The body is witness to the erasing and overwriting of times.' For Atkin, chronic illness is not merely an alternative temporality but a revelation that time *has no* absolute reality. Chronic illness

> reveals the folded nature of time. The arbitrary nature of time. It shows us time as experiential, not as we agree to pretend it is: not linear, not progressive, not leading from one moment to the next and the next and so on, but all at once, a pile up of time, a mess of time. ... Linear time loses meaning or substance. We see it for the cheap lie it is.[8]

What is striking here is that both this revelation and the experience of time which yields it are themselves apparently more painful than liberating. I think of the night mail worker again and how much clock time – however much it deceives that it is an objective metric, an invariable precondition of experience – is (for that very reason) still 'in' us all.

Resistance to linear representation of the experience of chronic illness perhaps also underestimates, therefore, the possibilities for 'self-definition' or 'self-concept' that an 'illness chronology' (as Charmaz calls it) can release:

> When illness serves as a timemarker, people use it as a major source of the stops, hurdles, highs and lows that give their lives shape and structure. Illness chronologies chart events, specify durations, and locate places and people. . . . [They render chronically ill people's] experiences more comprehensible . . . help them explain what happened, why they got worse or better and what illness meant to them.

Benchmarks in an illness chronology, that is to say, frame and define experience as much as physical symptoms or relative health and illness, providing 'windows for observing the developing self'. Events acquire significance because ill people view them 'as turning points that mirror growth . . . a more aware self and positive [and] changed involvements'. Importantly, 'markers are not merely reconstructions after the events'. While 'some timemarkers seem objective and external' (and often do not exist in the mind and memory of the ill person as we saw in Chapter 6), in contrast,

> identifying moments and significant events are existential. They touch the self directly. Identifying moments are telling moments filled with new self-images. And they are telling because they spark sudden realisations, reveal hidden images of self.[9]

This is an important reminder that personal stories of illness are by no means driven by clock time. Linear chronology, as here conceived, is subjective: 'turning points' are not objectively but existentially determined; narrative form has meaning according to inner logic and contours. The idea that progressive models of being are not incompatible with the kind of non-normative or present-centred experiences of time which chronic illness can foreground, and which operate outside of conventional health narratives, is a key one to which I return later in this chapter.

The chief reason I have floated non-narrative modes of practice and thinking at the start of this chapter, however, is because the originating and presiding emphases – on not using language and not using story – might seem (at least in part) incompatible with my emphasis on the value of literature, and on fictional narrative, as an intervention in the experience of pain. In fact, Wasson's enterprise is an affined literary one; and story and narrative do not alone, of course, comprise or represent literature. Furthermore, while the work of Padfield and Wasson together demonstrates how chronic pain exposes the limits of narrative which Woods highlights, both also show how pain engenders language and the need for its expression. Padfield was struck by how the co-creation of a photograph 'fed into the verbal as much as the visual dialogue': 'Focussing on visual objects and their juxtapositions, rather than verbal histories, changed the type of dialogue possible. Through the process of image-making, sufferers articulated, sometimes poetically, sometimes with alarming starkness, the conflicting and multi-faceted nature of pain.'[10] But the true source of affinity (as well as tension) with these ideas is actually a mutual concern with 'translating'[11] (the key verb of Wasson's project) the 'rich inner world'[12] (as Woods puts it) or the 'dark', 'primal space' which remains (says Padfield) otherwise 'unconscious' and 'unreachable'.[13] The final three reading case studies which follow are examples of both narrative and poetry at once *finding* such buried pain at its emotional source, and *representing* or 'speaking' it, in ways which cumulatively, as I shall demonstrate, throw a fresh perspective on the debate around the place and value of narrative in the alleviation of pain. In the course of detailing the case studies, I also begin gradually (though by no means entirely) to move away from the explanatory paradigms I have harnessed from the body of work around reading and psychology and gravitate further towards the support of psychoanalysis, the science of the pain of primal emptiness (to use Padfield's words) as we saw in Chapter 1. Gendlin, with a foothold in both camps, as it were, provides the intellectual bridge.

Susan

In this session, there are only three members present. The group size fluctuated owing to the limitations on attendance variously caused by the group members' pain conditions, their medical appointments or their family responsibilities. Nevertheless, the group was unusually small (six or seven was the average weekly number). The group members I concentrate on here – Susan (a mother in her forties) and Deborah (a young woman in her twenties whose overall medical condition worsened considerably during the course of the study) – have figured in some of the sessions discussed already, and they, like Michael (the third member present and the subject of the final case study below), were among the most regular attendees. The group is reading Laurie Sheck's short poem 'Mysteriously Standing'.

'This looks heavy', says Susan, as she glances at the poem ahead of the group leader's reading of it. When the first reading has concluded, there is a significantly extended silence, as group members continue to look thoughtfully at the poem. 'Sorry', explains Deborah, 'I had to read that again'. At the group leader's request, Deborah proceeds to read the poem again, aloud, to the group. There is another (shorter) silence, then:

> *Michael [looking at the poem the whole time]:'These intervals of withdrawal where I am a burned field/And above me the sky is thickening . . .'[14] Could it be someone describing – how maybe – something without feeling – [looking up now, smiling faintly, glancing around at the others, as if to appeal to their patience] – how something that you – you don't think has feelings might feel? The feelings of something that can't feel. That sounds unusual doesn't it? (looking for signs of understanding of what he has said)*
>
> *Susan: A burned field – sometimes you see farmers burning the old crop off, don't you? So a burnt field is where a farmer leaves it to – regrow – to – re-energise the soil for next year's crop.*
>
> *Michael:Could you put it in the person – sort of describing the way they're feeling?*
>
> *Susan:You're burnt out –*
>
> *Deborah:But the sky's thickening above you so it's like [hand reaches to head in deep thought, eyes on poem] feeling stormy and empty at the same time. [Quietly] I – I can – I can see myself in this poem definitely. When I've withdrawn it is because I'm [shakes head] empty, I'm done, I'm exhausted. I've given everything I can give. You're kind of switched off. And I've got to kind of – come out – take time, and then come back in – to life, into the world.*
>
> *Susan:You withdraw totally 'cause you're physically and mentally drained [hands imitate something being pulled or pouring from her body], and you just can't do it anymore. It's as if your body and brain withdraw for you when you get to the edge. When you're under so much stress, you just have to take yourself away from it for a little while.*

> *Group Leader:Spent – you've given all –*
> *Micahel:Left like – barren.*
> *Susan: I am a burned field' – that's a really really **really** good way of*
>   *describing yourself sometimes isn't it?*

The mode of literary-stylistic variation known as foregrounding has been shown, as we have seen, to be associated with increased reading times and greater affect, responses that are apparently independent of literary competence or experience.[15] This instance of in vivo reading by relatively inexperienced readers is not merely corroborative of this finding, as the group members (at first individually) dwell on and grapple with the poem's difficulty in silent and vocal re-readings. The unfamiliarity of the poetic language also produces an unusual dislocation in the reader's own usage: *Could it be . . . how maybe – something without feeling – how something that you – how something that you – you don't think has feelings might feel?*. Michael's disrupted syntax is symptomatic of an effort to give substance to *something* not there (***without** feeling*) – something that is nonetheless real – in an intense struggle analogous to the poem's own creative endeavour. 'Foregrounding', to recall Mukařovský, 'is the *opposite* of automization'[16] (my emphasis). What is interesting here is that deautomatization is demonstrable not only in the disturbance of normal speech patterns in Michael's formulation but also in the use of language that is 'everyday' (the very communication which, as we saw in Chapter 5, foregrounding deliberately disrupts[17]). When Susan says of the poem's central metaphor '*that's a really really **really** good way of describing yourself sometimes*', there is a '*re-energised*' life (to use Susan's own word) that is wholly absent from the suffering which Susan powerfully recognizes in the image and is even now re-feeling (*at the edge*) in response to the poem. Rather than simply or singly thinking what a terrible thing this is to be, Susan is thinking what a good way this is of describing it! Both Michael's and Susan's responses are as far as they could be, moreover, from the tonal register of lack and subtraction which characterized the CBT sessions we have witnessed (*I can't, I don't*), even despite the emphatically painful feelings of incapacity that, triggered by the poem's language, are verbalized in this exchange: '*empty*', '*exhausted*', '*switched off*', '*drained*', '*spent*', '*barren*'. How *can* this be so '*really really **really** good*' – and the whole session (to an onlooker and as verified by group members at interview) has this feel and atmosphere – when it ought to be so bad?

Gendlin describes the 'feeling' of authentically articulating experience thus:

To conceptualise a feeling in words that really seem to convey it . . . makes the feeling more intense, more clear, more real, and more capable of being handled. The client feels as if they now know where, in them, it is to be found. They feel as if they had grappled with it and now own it, instead of being dogged by something partly unknown.

Moreover, 'the effect of saying it in therapy occurs via the experiencing of what is said':

> People have always fallen into the trap of interpreting their experience through stereotyped concepts whereby the actual stream of experience is largely missed. [When an individual is referring directly to their experiencing] not the verbal *content* but the *kind of process* occurring, will determine whether . . . they are *merely* using words, or whether their words are part of a deeper process. What their words are *about* will not tell us this.[18]

So, for example, with Susan's '*really really* **really** *good*': felt sense, authentic life, deep process, can be located in verbalization that is far from conventionally novel or creative. Nonetheless, it is the difficult, unfamiliar *literary* language (not that of 'therapy') which 'finds' the feeling; and the saying of it is first 'experienced' through the medium of the words of the poem.

At the interview, Susan explained that she had suffered a severe breakdown twelve months previously as a result of losing, in succession, her health, her job, her partner and her house (home, for nineteen years, to herself and her three grown-up children).

> *You just can't see it at the time. You don't know where you are going to turn. I had lost who I was. There would be days I wouldn't get up, times I wouldn't shower or dress. I never used to be like this. I was always a strong person leading a very active life in work – in everything. To be struck down like this, it's just – unnatural for me. I am still not strong.*

Of the reading group experience, Susan said:

> *These sessions helped me a lot. Because I compartmentalise things that have happened to me in the past. We have been through these experiences, me and my children. We talk about it and then it is put to one side, because I don't feel that it should be constantly talked about. Nobody knows what has gone on inside of me. But to bring it out like that [points to the poem]. Maybe it's a way of expressing something that I – an alternative way – because I have experienced a feeling like this but I don't know how many other people may or may not have experienced that sort of situation. So is it normal? Is it not normal? What I mean is, it's a way of expressing it without having to tell people, if that makes sense?*

'Nobody knows what has gone on inside of me.' But the *text*, Susan found, somehow did. This intensely visual poem is like a verbal equivalent of the photographs in Padfield's study, at once 'connecting to an unconscious pre-verbal part' of self while 'translating that part into an objective "readable" object'.[19] Of a client who was able verbally to grapple with her suffering, Gendlin said: '[Before] her bad feelings were diffused throughout her body. Her whole body hurt. But now she had localised the problem . . . the rest of her body was released.'[20] Instead of being 'dogged by something partly unknown',[21] 'the whole body is alive in a less constricted way'.[22] Significantly, the pain consultants in this study came to the same conclusion in explaining why the reading group helped to decrease the pain for days afterwards. *I think they're better able to deal with it as just pain rather than as global suffering. The rest of the week, even though the pain is bad, they're less distressed by it. Some of the patients I know through the clinic seem much more well after [prolonged exposure to] Shared Reading than they were before. There's fluctuation of course but that's against a background of lesser suffering.* Perhaps connected to this is the fact that the poem's language also offered a mode of serious expression for something which, Susan felt, was *too* serious (and too upsetting for her children) for expression most of the time or in the rest of her life. *I don't feel that it should be constantly talked about.* Susan did not want to 'tell her story' in the conventional sense and would have resisted any call to do so, not least because her experience did not permit of simple or straightforward telling: *You just can't see . . . you don't know.* But she emphatically does not resist – quite the contrary – the power of the poem to discover and express her deep inner trouble without diminishment of its reality. Padfield recounts how one chronic pain sufferer, who chose to photograph her arm where cuts from self-harm were visible ('that is what the pain made me do', she said, 'it was the only way I could express it at the time'), found that it was only seeing the photograph of her arm, rather than her arm itself, which 'made me realise what I had done to myself'.[23] Analogously, the poem's imagery enables Kate not only to 'realise' or (in Gendlin's term) 'own' her feeling. It also allows her to *keep* it as her own (*a way of expressing it without having to tell people*), a private witness of meaning.

Deborah

At the time this session took place, Deborah was in the process of appealing against a catastrophic change in her benefit eligibility, even as her physical capacity was deteriorating, which had left her without means to leave the house independently. Deborah described herself as usually *a glass half full type of person: Life has knocked me down, flat on my face a few times, and I've built myself back up and say, 'Right, well I can't do this, so I will go and do that then. If that path is barred, I can go and find a new one'.* She admitted that she was struggling, more than ever before, at this time, to find a new path, *to get back up and get back to me:*

> *The times you are in a very deep depression, you go, you go far away not just from the people that you love, but from yourself, who you are. You become quite a different person. You can hold so many thoughts in your head – the words just aren't there. It is hard to explain something – that there is not words for.*

The group is *useful*, Deborah said, *because it gets out thoughts that would otherwise stay inside.* On hearing herself re-read the Laurie Sheck poem at the interview, Deborah said: *There have been times when I've felt a little bit overcome when I've been reading out loud. That quiver in my voice* [at 'In that field, little Stonehenge of the heart'[24]], *I felt it – the words – as I was reading it.* What touched Deborah in this line unfolded into explicitness later in the reading session:

> *Michael:It's like a kind of a feeling that's been there for a long, long time.*
> *Deborah: And maybe the heart is Stonehenge because – because*
>   *maybe you're protecting that heart [pauses and folds one curled hand*
>   *inside the other, looking intently at the group leader who is nodding*
>   *encouragingly] by withdrawing for a little bit. It's so that you are*
>   *'uninjured' – still standing – you've kind of switched off and withdrawn*
>   *temporarily, and because you've done that, it's not permanent.*
> *Susan: And you can see the 'Light'* [the central word of the poem which
>   begins a new line]
> *Deborah: I thought that was strange how 'Light' kind of went across the*
>   *line. It's a strange placing.*
> *Group Leader: How would it be if it was on the same line instead of*
>   *'Mysteriously standing, its distinct construction odd and injured in this*
>   *yellow/Light'.*[25]
> *Deborah: It's like the light's separate from the withdrawal isn't it? It does*
>   *really separate the two. It comes – after. [Using her fingers to imitate*
>   *the separation as she looks up, smiling.]*

Deborah's words and facial expression have the force of 'conviction', in the sense in which Freud uses the term: to refer to an indication of assent which 'seems to arise spontaneously and appear unbidden'[26] when the analyst communicates to the analysand an understanding (interim and incomplete) put together from the 'fragments' or 'traces' left behind by repressed material. 'This can be translated without any hesitation into: "Yes, you're right this time – about my unconscious".[27] Deborah's smile is just such a 'yes', an 'indirect confirmation' as to the poem's intuitively feeling 'right' or 'fitting in' with her own psychic processes. But it is as if the poem gives not an interpretation, but a syntax. Unlike the analyst's constantly modified reflection of the 'fresh material pouring in',[28] the poem stays the same insofar as the words on the page are permanent. But the surprise of that *strange placing* is new and fresh every time the poem is read. Deborah's *feeling* the words and lines as she reads, repeats at once the poem's structural-emotional dynamic and (in miniature) her own psychological one of withdrawal and *coming back in to life, to the world.* She said, as part of this exchange: *To varying degrees you could go through this process many times a day even. Or at certain times you might go very far away. And stay there a long time. That field might be left fallow for a while, before it's built back up again.* But the process is not, here and now, something suffered 'inside' which 'stays' there, untranslated into thought. It is 'out' there in the language of the poem. Or, rather, there is no 'in' versus 'out' here, but, as the syntactic contours of the poem's emotion touch off what is deep within Deborah, there are two powerfully resonating *insides.* 'Meaning', says Gendlin, 'is *formed* in the interaction of experiencing and [concept]. . . . We cannot even know what a concept "means" or use it meaningfully without the "feel" of its meaning. No amount of symbols, definitions and the like can be used in the place of the *felt* meaning'.[29] Poetry, as we see it in operation in Deborah – as in Susan – is demonstrably where concept and experiencing, feeling and meaning, are at one. Moreover, 'by the time we say exactly what we meant it isn't quite the same: it is richer, more explicit, more fully known. . . . It specifies it, adds to it, goes beyond it . . . in short, *changes* it'.[30] The poetry does not merely reflect, it transforms, because knowing, owning, *having* an emotional experience is the key change. This is Bion's territory of course, and I return to it shortly.

It is noteworthy that, at the moment of this happening – in the reading session itself – there is not a narrative in sight, neither a literary nor a personal one. For a person whose inner trouble is too deep or hardened for ready access, it is the struggle for expression that is more palpable than an available personal story. Here it is the poetic language – a single word, line or image – which initiates and aids that process by first reaching the deep inner trouble that needs expression, even where the person might be wholly unaware of that need. But the next and final case study shows why it might finally be misleading to regard poetry – atemporal, fragmentary, episodic – as *more* therapeutic than (literary) story in the sense of giving representative form.

Michael

Michael is a married man in his forties, a father, with a career background in public service. From the outset of reading Bowen's short story, 'The Visitor', Michael was notably attuned to the child's state of mind. 'Here was he alone, enisled with tragedy.'[31] *'Enisled' – what does that mean? Is it like full?* Michael asks of the group leader. *Well I suppose*, she replies, *I'm seeing it as being separated off in some way, like an island.* Michael nods: *That's what made me think like full of tragedy, like you're filled with it, like there's nothing else.* When the group leader reads, 'Roger had never believed that the Miss Emerys or any of the people he and his mother visited really went on existing after one had said good-bye to them and turned one's back',[32] Michael again gently nods his head, saying thoughtfully, *It's because you can't – can't comprehend when you're a child that other people can be doing things that you can't see.*

> *Group Leader: It's funny when he says he knew with his brain that people went on like their clocks but he didn't believe it. You'd think that knowing with your brain would be more proof or more real than believing in something, but he knows it in his brain yet doesn't believe it.*
>
> *Michael: Well, that's because he's very young isn't it and he can't – can't fully reason the way things work. He's in a bit of a daydream as well. It says [returning to a sentence earlier in the passage] 'The thing had crouched beside his bed all night; he had been conscious of it through the thin texture of his dreams. He reached out again now, timidly, irresistibly to touch it, and found that it had slipped away'.[33] It's like – his thoughts are involved with imagination and the thoughts may not be real – it's like a mixture. [Leaning forward intently, eyes resting now on his hands, now making contact with the group leader, speaking slowly and carefully, concentrating hard.] When a child's thinking about something or about somebody else, what they're thinking may not be real or not really happening. He knows someone is going to die, it's going to happen. But he still can't be sure what's real and what's imaginary. I think it's sort of like being in a kind of shock isn't it? When something bad happens, sometimes you just can't believe it. I came off a motorbike once. It seemed like it was in slow motion. It's like it's not really happening to you, it's like a dream. Even though it's really slow, you still can't stop what's happening to you. And of course, he's just a child. The loss of the mother is going to be a great big thing in his little life.*

In this final utterance (*a great big thing*), Michael unconsciously recalls and reuses the words he has just now quoted from the text ('The *thing* had crouched beside his bed all night').

When the group resumes their reading of the story, the boy, still awaiting the news he doesn't want to receive, hears a clock tick out in the passageway:

> It had no expression in its voice, neither urged one nor restrained one, simply commented quite impartially upon the flight of time. Sixty of these ticks went to make a minute, neither more nor less than sixty, and the hands of the clock would be pointing to an hour and a minute when they came to tell Roger what he was expecting to hear. Round and round they were moving, waiting for that hour to come.[34]

Fay: It's unusual for a child to notice how slowly the fingers are moving on the clock. [Fay mimics the clock hand using her own, performing a slow arc in the air. Michael listens intently, then stares ahead and brings his hand to his face in deep thought.]

Group Leader: Unless they're very bored or lonely or something. Sometimes my grandma used to fix watches and clocks and it would be tick tick tick all around. There was nothing to do there so you were kind of drawn into listening to them.
    [As the group enjoy the anecdote, Michael moves his arm directly forward onto the table. His extended hand, on its side, straight and pointed, is moving gently backwards and forwards.]
Michael: I used to look at the clock when I was a child and try to will [hand moves up and down in the same place] the second hand to stop. [Laughs quietly to himself.]
Group Leader: Why, was that because of something you didn't want to happen?
Michel: (very quietly) Yes. [Michael withdraws his arm, half-covers his face with his hand, and closes his eyes, no longer smiling.]
Group Leader [as the group members, one by one, look back down at the text]: Yeah, yeah . . . yeah, that is, . . . do you think there's . . . does that feel . . . like there's something like that going on with him, the boy, do you think?

In the momentary silence which follows, or, more truly, *surrounds*, Michael's single word, 'yes', everyone present – the group leader (who struggles to recover), the group members who tactfully look down again at the text – all sense that Michael (so vocal up to this point in the session) is himself now 'enisled in tragedy'. It is a pause almost tangibly full of something amorphously unnameable: visibly too emotionally powerful to be fitted into words.

*

'Experiencing is an inward sensitivity of the living body . . . a physically felt "this" [to which we inwardly point]. It is what we inwardly "are", "mean" or "feel" at a given moment.'[35] If you are willing to think from experiencing, says Gendlin – from the preconceptual 'more', the unsayable 'excess', the vaguely felt edge of the implicit in the felt sense of a situation – if you 'attend to it directly':

> Then you can notice that it will not permit you to say most of the cogent things you can easily say. It will stay . . . stuck and mum unless and until just certain sentences 'come' to open it. . . . What you find is not disorder, not limbo. . . . Rather, you find an intricacy, pregnant, implicitly ordered, perhaps partly opaque. From this intricacy you may at times be unable to go on, at least for a while.[36]

Michael's barely uttered 'Yes', the instinctive shrinking, as it were, into his own body which accompanies the word, bespeaks just such a moment of stuckness – pregnant yet inarticulate, intricate yet opaque – where something subterranean, some residuum of experience seems unconsciously to seek a form of realization which eludes it. It is the kind of happening which the therapeutic process is always in search of.

> All therapy [is] a working with inner experiencing. It is a process of inner grappling. . . . The individual in psychotherapy struggles with many experiences that he or she has never symbolised before and for which he or she knows no symbols. . . . Clients often report being 'disturbed', 'unsettled', 'churning', having 'something going on in them' but not knowing what.[37]

'Not knowing what'. In their famous conclusion, in *Studies in Hysteria*, that their patients 'suffer mainly from reminiscences', Freud and Breuer add: 'Recollection without affect almost invariably produces no result. The psychical process which originally took place must be repeated as vividly as possible; it must be brought back to its status nascendi and then given verbal utterance.'[38] The moment of disturbance, unsettlement, churn we witness in Michael here is the effect not of therapy, nor (simply) of recollection *with* affect. What the moment of reading finds here is indistinguishable from the 'status nascendi' of an original pain.

*

Michael witnessed this moment on a video-recording at interview. (There are two related passages her which I label A and B for ease of reference.)

A.

At that minute I feel a little bit upset. I felt as though I wanted to cry. I think maybe I had some understanding of how the child felt because I remember how I felt [lengthy pause]. I suppose it was completely different to the situation in the story but sometimes things unlock – open certain doors, those doors to maybe old memories that you – you prefer to keep locked shut. He didn't want to know. He would rather have those doors shut.

The shifts in pronoun use are striking here. ***I** wanted to cry; old memories that* **you – you** *prefer to keep shut.* The shift to 'you' has long been recognized in reading research as indicating that the reader is 'enacting the implications of the story for his or her own understanding, merging the identities of protagonist and self in a single, although complex, perspective'.[39] The process of 'merging' and the perspective thereby released is complex indeed in that final shift of pronoun: ***He** didn't want to know.* ***He** would rather have those doors shut.* Behind the *He* is Michael's sustained immersion on first reading, now reawakened at this revisiting of the story, in the boy's sense of loneliness and shock. A little later in the interview, Michael talked of the trauma of being subject to a long period of abuse when he was young:

B.

The way things were when I was a child. Everything was a secret really. I was just locked into what was going on and in a dream world and I suppose the dream world part of it was like an escape from the reality of what was actually going on at that time. And probably I felt safer being in a dream world and I probably didn't want to know. I didn't really want to know what was happening to me.

Michael, as a child, found himself, like the boy, continuously and passively caught between two *worlds* whose reality he doubted: the *dream* world to which he escaped and the *actual* world in which he was *locked*, a world so *secret* as not to qualify as reality for anybody else. In Passage A, then, ***He*** (*He didn't want to know*) is also a version of ***I*** (*I remember how I felt*). And this ***I*** is not itself singular but at once doubled *and* merged. Both Michael-adult ('I remember') and Michael-child ('I felt') are implicated at this moment. 'Past experience does not function in the present as the discrete events that have happened in the past', says Gendlin. 'All the past and all the complex aspects of myself today can be involved in the experiencing of my telling the incident. They can be here now to be worked with.'[40] This is a Freudian axiom, of course: 'We need to treat the illness not as a matter belonging to the past, but as a force operating in the present. . . . While the patient experiences it as something intensely real and immediate, it is our job to do the therapeutic work.'[41] Likewise, the therapeutic value of literary reading in this instance is not just its unwilled retrieval of specific autobiographical memory but its putting the reader, Michael, involuntarily in place and in touch with what is unresolved in past experience. A further symptomatic trace of this past-present conjunction is Michael's telling and moving substitution of personal pronouns within parallel syntax across the two testimonies above, one relating to the literary narrative (*He* *didn't want to know.* *He* *would rather have those doors shut,* Passage A), one to his own story (*I* *probably didn't want to know.* *I* *didn't really want to know what was happening to me,* Passage B).

At the close of the interview, the researcher said: *I am just thinking that those two things, the chronic pain and the trauma of the abuse, they are both sort of hidden things aren't they? Yes*, Michael said. *No one can ever see them.*

Michael's disclosure in the post-group interview gave retrospective power to this moment from the final session of the study, where the group was reading the conclusion to *Of Mice and Men*. Lennie, the childlike man, has inadvertently killed the wife of his employer and is fleeing the scene:

It was very quiet in the barn, and the quiet of the afternoon was on the ranch. . . . A pigeon flew in through the open hay door and circled and flew out again. . . . As happens sometimes, a moment settled and hovered and remained for much more than a moment. And sound stopped and movement stopped for much, much more than a moment.[42]

Michael: We're left looking at that feeling, that atmosphere in the barn. That's the feeling Lennie has got inside himself. With the pigeon flying in and the advance of day – it's showing you that life goes on. Nature just going about its daily business. Life continuing as it normally does. People saying hello and going about their lives as if this bad thing hasn't happened. Lennie must be feeling this can't be true, it can't be real. [Visibly struggling to find the words as the group leader notices.]
Group Leader: He knows everything's changed forever. But the rest of the world doesn't. You can't quite believe the world's carrying on.

> *Michael: They could be talking to you and you don't hear a word they're saying. You could see the world going on as normal but what had happened to you might feel unbelievable, you know, hard to accept.*

Michael (amid the shift in pronouns – *we*, *he*, *you*) is attuned to two distinct inward experiences here: on the one hand, the feeling that trauma leaves behind *inside*; on the other hand, the further trauma produced by having to carry on, *with* that inside, as though one were just the same. *The pain is still there*, said Michael at the interview, *locked away inside.*

*

'We can only find a way to enter into the making and breaking of narrative in clinical settings if we attend first to what is unfinished, incomplete and tentative – the myriad forms of "nonnarrative" communication, including all the dimensions of embodied interaction'.[43] Manifestly, narrative has every inch the power of poetry to 'enter into' or attend to the 'unfinished' in experience, which slips story per se. Indeed, as we have seen, it is the specific properties of *literary* narrative that foster this attention; involuntarily stimulating 'expressive enactment'; taking on or bringing into presence 'the embodied perspective of a textual other'; and experiencing, at the level of deeply 'felt sense', the 'affective resonance between personal memories and the world of the text'.[44] This is where, as Woods points out, it is essential not to collapse distinctions between different narrative forms and contexts. 'Emphasising the continuities between, for example, hospital anecdotes, published autobiographies and diagnostic interviews, diverts attention away from systemic analysis of the diverse functions and effects of specific types of storytelling.'[45]

More importantly, this case study centres on the tensions that have frequently crossed this section of the book between clock and chronic time, and between linear and lived narrative. It seems no coincidence that the key passage from Bowen's story is concerned with the minute workings of an authoritative timepiece ('It must be a very big one. Perhaps a station master's clock'). Roger is super-sensitized to the clock's 'ticking-out'. He hears its steady measuring precision as an expressionless 'voice', just as (and while) he 'expect[s] to **hear**' news of his mother's death. He feels in his own body, that is to say, how clock time's 'impartial', blank indifference is both in and out of time with that exact hour and minute to which the young boy's deepest emotional life is already mortgaged, ahead of the clock hand's pointing to it, in 'waiting for that hour to come'.[46] Two orders of time, two cosmologies, in one small child.

I suggested in Chapter 6 that the reading of literature offers an alternative temporality which shares affinity with, and is potentially experientially in tune with, 'crip' time or chronic (illness) time. Like crip time, literary time 'has the power to extract us from linear, progressive time'.[47] It is a space in which to re-imagine, or alternatively experience, or tangentially exist within, the present (as well as the contemporary) moment, free from the strictures of institutionalized time, whether this is conceived as medical-scientific, capitalist-economic, epistemological-ideological or as the austere condition of an individual life. As a Shared Reading group leader in a women's prison put it, the literary work presents, in every sense, 'a temporary life we happen to find ourselves in, that both is and is not ours'.[48] This is no negligible consideration if we are to take seriously the claim, as witnessed in Chapter 1, that the pathological temporal imperatives of Western modernity are responsible for the current epidemics of chronic sickness. Literary time's emancipatory potentials are bound up with its therapeutic ones. And it is possible, as I have suggested, that the lived experience of chronic or crip time, which the members of the chronic pain reading group share in common, encourages a predisposition, or susceptibility, to literature's temporal dismantlings.

Nonetheless, Michael's reading experience and the relation to buried pain it helped disclose do not speak in favour of prioritizing a present-centred, fragmentary, episodic self-experience, *in place*, or *at the expense*, of narrative accounting. As Gendlin says, the past is always *in* the present of experiencing – albeit often in a more volatile and potentially more accessible way for those living with chronic illness – and therein lies the therapeutic opportunity. 'A moment's experiencing contains implicitly so many meanings . . . the whole life of the person as it occurs in this present. . . . All areas of the personality are involved (and can change) in any one moment's experiencing even though verbally just some small meaning is thought or spoken.'[49] However small and fragmentary the meaning, a whole life! all the personality! can be transformed. The happening is of the present, but its implications are not. Therapeutic intervention is always fundamentally premised upon the cooperative tension between present reality (the moment in therapy) and life lived in time (growth, maturity, learning from experience). In a case study of treating a patient with chronic mental illness, who over the course of eighteen months progressed from frequent hospitalization to assisted living, Sebastian von Peter draws on Husserl's notion of the 'extended now' to describe the present of the therapeutic encounters which resulted in decisive change over the course of the treatment:

The present obtains a spatial extension . . . is allowed its own thickness and temporal spread, imagined as a three-dimensional network, encompassing and integrating the past and future. Instead of conceiving of a fleeting punctual now in the form of a 'knife-edge' present, the present [is] thought of as a temporally extended field . . . emerging out of all tenses. . . . [It is] an eventful space, recombining various events, feelings, thoughts and decisions, and inherently creative and productive . . . a flexible matrix . . . modifiable in different ways and from different directions.

What we have witnessed across Part II, I suggest, is how the present of literary reading is just such an 'eventful space', or crucible for change. Von Sebastian calls this 'creative time', distinguished, in his description, from both the notion of time as 'an absolute category', 'an objective and universal measure', and from present time as fragmentary, 'vanishing':

> [Its] temporal logic contrasts with the conception of the present as a mere fleeting sequence of now-points, focussing on moments of sheer disappearance. . . . Instead the notion of the extended now has to be perceived as the very embodied matrix from which a person is composed.[50]

I return in Chapter 10 and at the close of this book to the special significance of the 'creative' present for people living with chronic illness as well as to the related notion of 'readiness', or changing 'in their own time', which the pain consultants raised in Chapter 7.

For now, at the close of this chapter, I come back to the other aspect of this debate in relation to linear and present extension; the relative value, that is, of modes of representation (narrative, poetic, visual). I propose that what is really at stake in these reading moments is not the specific form they take but the degree to which they *find* or *constitute* form – how far they answer, that is, what Howard Levine calls the 'representational imperative': the 'demand upon the mind' exerted by emotional turbulence, for psychic work 'to transform the previously unspeakable', make it 'thinkable'.[51] The pressure of this psychic demand first commences in what Bion calls an 'impingement',[52] summoning and activating an effort of awareness to give what is unspoken or unfinished, definition and tangible reality. In Michael's 'Yes', or in the quiver in Deborah's reading voice, the impingement is the action of the literary text as it provokes the sudden retrieval of deep personal matter, seeking expression, however minimal and strugglingly inarticulate, in order not to be merely hidden, lost or forgotten. 'Representation of the previously unrepresentable . . . is a lifelong, homeostatic task in which the inherently traumatic sensations of being alive and suffering are contained, ameliorated and made somewhat more tolerable.'[53] For people living with pain, the need for such a 'vital protective'[54] function is arguably as chronic as the condition itself. I propose in what follows, on the basis of the illustrative evidence of the foregoing reading examples, that literary reading is especially well placed to help with this lifelong task.

*

At its most basic level, literary reading involves unforced practice in inner thinking (akin, though at a more fundamental level, to its offering an alternative to programmatic training in autobiographical memory as we saw in Chapter 6). Encouraging the growth or activation of commensurate containers for the richness and depth of thoughts and feelings derived from emotional experience has become, as we saw in Part I, the primary aim of psychoanalytic therapy, following Bion. The goal is particularly pressing and necessary for psychoanalysts such as Levine, who encounter versions of alexithymia frequently in their work. 'I have found', he says,

> that with these patients a good deal of the analytic process and the work of the cure revolves around the analyst's role not only in uncovering and helping them to discover . . . unacceptable but hidden aspects of themselves, but in strengthening and developing their capacities for representation. It is the very capacity to think that is at issue.

Creating the very 'instruments for thinking' is essential to give people emotional relief from the 'pressures that arise from inchoate feeling states that are not yet structured, bound or specified by attachment to words'. Without the ability to achieve stable psychic representation of emotional reality, individuals are left susceptible, as we saw in Part I, to 'fears of engulfment' and 'terror of confronting the emptiness or void': Bion's nameless dread. In these circumstances, the analyst's role is less to discover and decode hidden meaning or a pre-existent narrative than to 'initiate' or 'catalyse'[55] processes and potentially transformative movements which enable the analysand to give form to something that was previously weakly represented. This process, says Levine, is inherently intersubjective and co-creative. The emphasis is on naming and describing feeling states or affective experiences emerging from the emotional interaction, relationship and reality between analyst and patient, such that meaning is 'shaped and assembled moment to moment'[56] from the affective context in which it occurs. The role of the analyst is to 'be open to and to absorb' a patient's internal reality allowing it to 'sojourn' [Bion's word][57] 'within the psyche and personhood of the analyst long enough . . . to be worked on by the analyst's alpha function and transformed into something that can be either *thought with* or *thought about* by the analyst'. The co-construction of meaningful thoughts with and for the patient is more intuitive than deductive, based on 'internal emotional resonance', and 'unconscious, spontaneous participation in an active intersubjective process', as if the analyst were an 'alter ego'[58] who lends the capacity to think experience on another's behalf.

It is by no means a new idea to draw a parallel between the creative processes of the writer and those of the psychoanalyst.[59] But it is worth pointing out their unmistakable overlap in Levine's description of the psychoanalytic encounter:

'feeling or imagining what the patient may not yet clearly feel or know [with the effect of] helping to create or approximate something that may not yet have achieved sufficient presence in a figured form'.[60] Significantly, Thomas Ogden, psychoanalyst and novelist, calls the psychoanalytic process as advocated by Bion a form of self-renunciation, in terms which recall Keatsian or Lawrentian relinquishing of the artistic ego: 'the act of allowing oneself to become less definitively oneself in order to create a psychological space in which analyst and patient may enter into a shared state of intuiting and being at one with a disturbing psychic reality that the patient, on their own, is unable to bear'.[61] As Bion put it, 'The more "real" the psychoanalyst is the more he *can be at one* with the reality of his patients'[62] (my emphasis). For crucially, what at-one-ment entails for Bion is not simply or primarily enabling the co-creation of a container but, more riskily and essentially, *co-experiencing* the *contained.* 'When as psychoanalysts we are concerned with the reality of the personality there is more at stake than an exhortation to "know thyself, accept thyself, be thyself". . . . The point at issue is "being" that which is "real" . . . the real self, being O.' 'O' was how Bion denoted the ultimate reality 'of anything whatever',[63] – the really real, the Kantian thing-in-itself – precisely so as to capture its resistance to formal knowing. The analyst 'cannot know the O', but 'can only "be" it'.[64] Moreover, 'what the patient is saying and what the interpretation is', Bion suggested, in an apparently paradoxical statement, 'is in a sense relatively unimportant. Because by the time you are able to give [an interpretation] which the patient understands, all the work has been done'.[65]

This is the 'work', to put it in Gendlin's terms, of 'feeling meaning': 'The attempt, made by some clients, therapists and individuals generally to *replace* the experiencing by use of explanations will neither really explain nor change anything. If we do not have the felt meaning of the concept, we haven't got the concept at all, only a verbal noise. Nor can we *think* without felt meaning.'[66] The concept or container – the interpretation or holding explanation – is at once necessary *and* secondary, essential *and* provisional, the apparent end *and* the mere means. The further (seeming) paradox is that the interpretation when it comes might be as creatively emergent or 'imagined' as the process which produces it and (so far as simple fact is concerned) a relative fiction. 'Rather than certainties, we are often – perhaps always – left to some extent with beliefs, hypotheses, speculations, plausible theories. . . . Rather than uncovering and naming repressed hard factual truths that correspond to historical reality, our interpretations are often constructions.'[67] The specific finalized form which the emotional reality takes is not predetermined, but one of the emergent possibilities that feels fitting and unique, personalized and subjectivized, even as it will be contingent upon and carry the emotional imprint of the moment and its specific quality of attunement and at-one-ment. For the priority is not factual but *emotional* truth, not preconceived but *vital* form. The goals are 'to say something that feels both true to the emotional experience of any given moment of an analytic session, and that is utilizable by the analytic pair for psychological work'.[68] What is said needs to be capable of thus being 'used' by the analysand to form meanings 'which resonate with emotions in relation to which the patient can increasingly afford to feel more alive without the need to split them off or deaden himself to them'.[69] The exchange must give the patient 'a feeling of existence, in which sufficient space can be formed . . . for their silent self and where [meaning] can be acquired without there being a compression of their inner world'.[70]

I contend that it is just such 'a feeling of existence' and 'alive' emotionally resonant meaning that we have witnessed in the reading group members across this chapter. I speculate further that literature is potentially so powerful an ally of psychoanalysis because psychoanalysis is in many ways a derivation of the literary process: inhabiting truth at a primary level, and acting as its expressive witness. Significantly, in *Transformations*, Bion's own examples of O are literary-religious ones: Milton's *Paradise Lost* and the dark night of the soul in St John of the Cross. He also compares psychoanalytic transformations to artistic ones:

> The painter by virtue of his artistic capacity is able to transform . . . the original experience, the realisation [a landscape] into a painting (the representation). . . . By analogy with the artist . . . I propose that the work of the psychoanalyst should be regarded as transformation of a realisation (the actual psychoanalytic experience) into an interpretation or series of interpretations.[71]

What the case studies we've seen suggest, however, is that there is potentially more than analogy at stake between literary and psychoanalytic realizations, insofar as the literary text potentially offers a very unique kind of container. In these reading instances, there is a palpable sense of three things happening at once. An inner reality is accessed or touched off by the text: at the same time, the poem or story bears witness to that inner pain, is at-one with it; simultaneously, the literary work releases the pain into representation, tangible form, with an existence in time and place. It is catalyst and representation, contained and container, being and knowing, beta and alpha, experiencing and meaning. Aside from this manifold happening, nothing is predictable. The poem or story might or might not summon this activity or activate buried pain; there is no saying to whom it will happen or not happen; if it does touch off some inner content, the plasticity with which it might do so in the singular encounter between text and individual is as inexhaustible as the potential in literature itself, across its diversity of cultures and ages, to meet individual needs. If one poem or story doesn't work, the next one might:

something almost certainly will. And this process is potentially as continuous as experiencing itself.

Furthermore, literature does not fall foul of the 'first distortion of truth in the analytic situation . . . that it is an interaction between a sick person and a healthy one',[72] when, in truth, each brings their own psychological needs, dependencies and pathological defences. The literary text does not purport to be well or healthy. On the contrary, said D. H. Lawrence, famously, 'One sheds one's sicknesses in books, repeats and presents again one's emotions, to be master of them'.[73] What literature gives is the rawness of emotion and experience, *and* the possibility of mastery over them, again and again.

9

Shared reading and intersubjectivity: The group

Here at the conclusion of this section of the book, I turn to consider a key aspect of the reading encounters which I have only touched upon in passing thus far. Literary reading in this model takes place in a shared group setting. Thus, the intersubjectivity with the literary text, as demonstrated in the last chapter, is paralleled or extended through the intersubjectivity of group members with one another. My intention in this chapter is to disclose some of the key dynamics at play here as well as to explicate their therapeutic influence. The first section of the chapter, consistent with the orientation of much of this book, will consider Shared Reading in the light of Bion's early therapeutic work with groups, on which much of his later theory of thinking was founded. The latter part of the chapter will draw extendedly for the first time on the work of developmental psychoanalysis in order to probe more microscopically into aspects of the Shared Reading group process.

Bion and the 'work group'

Bion's experimental and pioneering work with groups began at the rehabilitation ward of Northfield Military Hospital and thereafter at the Tavistock clinic in the 1940s. The group task was to explore intra-group tensions (conflict, dependence, collaboration, self-interest) within the group itself, to study self-reflectively, that is, what the group members themselves were taking part in. Bion's approach was to 'establish no rules of procedure and put forward no agenda'. On the basis of this experience, Bion distinguished two types of 'group mentality'. The 'work group' mentality is one in which 'the capacity for cooperation . . . is great'. The work group '[mobilises] vigour and vitality' and 'certain ideas play a prominent part'. Above all, the idea and recognition of the need for 'development' is 'an integral part of it' as is 'the accepted validity of learning by experience', a key tenet of Bion's theory of thinking and the absence of which is fatal to growth.[1] As we saw in Chapter 4, it is (undigested emotional) experience which propels thinking, makes it necessary. 'Thinking is driven by the human need to know the truth – the reality of who one is and what is occurring in one's life' and 'the capacity for thinking is developed in order to come to terms with thoughts derived from one's disturbing emotional experience'. '[Only by means of] thinking that confronts reality in all its full unforgiving alterity . . . is it possible to do something with (to learn from and efficaciously attempt to modify) the reality of one's lived emotional experience.'[2] The work group mentality rises to this task, engaging in collaborative mental activity which wrestles with and contains emotional experience rather than discharging or evading it. 'It is almost as if human beings were aware of the painful and often fatal consequences of having to act without an adequate grasp of reality; and therefore were aware of the need for truth as a criterion in the evaluation of their findings.' But Bion came to recognize an unconscious dynamic whereby the group 'is unable to face the emotional tensions within it' and 'the situation is charged with emotions which exert a powerful, and frequently unobserved, influence on the group'. 'I am reminded of looking through a microscope at an overthick section: with one focus I see, not very clearly perhaps, but with sufficient distinctness, one picture. If I alter the focus very slightly I see another. . . . The picture of hard-working individuals striving to solve their psychological problems is displaced by a picture of a group mobilised to express its hostility and contempt' for the task at hand.

> Some contributions [a group member] is prepared to make as coming unmistakably from themselves, but there are others which they would wish to make anonymously. If the group can provide means by which contributions can be made anonymously, then the foundations are laid for a successful system of evasion and denial. . . . Each member [can] quite sincerely deny that they felt hostile.

This alternative mode of mental functioning is a means by which individuals pool emotions they wish to evade or deny. Unconsciously, these anonymized aspects of self become a collective entity – the group mentality – to which members are (hiddenly) collaboratively loyal and by which any hope of confronting painful emotional matter is (invisibly) prevented. 'Group mentality is the unanimous expression of the will of the group, contributed to by the individual in ways of which he or she is unaware.' It is constituted, Bion found, by unconscious commitment to one of three basic assumptions: the 'dependent' basic assumption is that the group leader will take on responsibility for the group tensions and the task of thinking; the 'pairing' mentality assumes that two members of the group will spawn a saving idea, or equivalent, that will rescue the group from the emotions it will not confront; the 'fight or flight' basic assumption is that the primitive or proto-matter the group fears can be dealt with by combating or running away from it. The basic assumption groups (as Bion called them) describe the 'group mentality', not the group members who commit to it; and as Bion's microscope analogy suggests, the focus can shift fluidly between the basic assumption and the work group mode. The important issue here is that basic assumption mentality is a threat to work group mentality and is developed to defend against the genuine thinking in relation to truth and reality in which it engages. Basic assumption groups obstruct, divert or dodge the dreaded 'questioning attitude' of the work group out of fear of emotional experiences 'for which [group members] do not feel prepared'.[3] Dependence on a selected person, on a pair or on fleeing or fighting is a means to oppose psychological work and to hide from knowledge, instead of achieving it. Basic group mentality is 'a jointly created anonymised form of anti-work', a 'conjoint compliance'[4] in anti-thinking.

Just as Bion applied his group experiences and analysis far beyond the psychoanalytic group,[5] so they are recognizable in the Shared Reading group study, though they are perhaps more immediately discernible, as might be expected, in the formally therapeutic CBT group. The evidence from the linguistic analysis applied to the transcripts of the CBT sessions found, for example, that a 'dependent' group culture was the default tendency: 'There is a clear distance between the coordinator and the participants. The coordinator is an out-group authority figure. He is constructed as expert and often dominates with expert knowledge.'[6] In Chapter 7, we caught a small but telling glimpse of how 'pairing' might be an alternative basic group assumption; when, that is, Holly and June, seated adjacently, spoke almost in unison about their position with regard to 'acceptance' of their chronic condition (Holly: *On a scale of 1–10 I'm probably at minus 10;* June: *Me, too*), while the rest of the group silently looked in their direction rather than at the group leader. At every level in this example, the group is unthreatened by the work group mentality and any painful feeling of change. Where Shared Reading is concerned, the orientation of the group is made more complex by the presence of the book as 'expert', as we shall see shortly. Moreover, the presence of the basic assumption mentality has been obscured thus far, because, in Part II, I have given almost exclusively examples of work group mentality in my quest to demonstrate how Shared Reading helps genuine thinking. Nonetheless, a fight/flight mentality was clearly evident as a response to the book or poem in various ways across all sessions. For example, on first reading Edwin Muir's poem, 'Dream and Thing' (which we encountered in Chapter 7), Susan told of how she had lost touch with her father when she was thirteen. *'My dream was to find him again. When I was eighteen, I found him and met up with him. My dream of what would be wasn't as good as what actually happened. He didn't really want to know.'* 'Don't like it', she said, pushing the poem away. This kind of outright emotional hostility was unusual and could be refocused (mindful of Bion's microscope analogy again) to form the basis of thinking work – as we saw with Fay in relation to 'The Visitor'. More often, fight or flight would take more banal forms of the kind Bion describes when he finds 'the group working together as a team . . . behaving as if we were equals, grown men and women, discussing the problem together freely, with tolerance for differences of opinion'.

> [When] the group has come together in this way it has become something as real and as much a part of human life as a family. [Yet] the group mentality [is] of such a nature that the needs of the individual [are] being successfully denied by the provision of a good friendly relationship between the patients [with the result that] mental activity becomes stabilised on a level that is platitudinous, dogmatic and painless. Development is arrested and the resultant stagnation is widespread.[7]

This is the kind of undemanding mentality which a Shared Reading group leader describes as dominating at certain points in any session. 'The continual initial challenge I encountered with the group was a recurrent inability to get anything primary or personal out of the text at points when we would pause from reading. The novel goes into emotional areas that often felt too hard to handle.'[8] There is an element of this resistance in the initial 'summary' or 'about' statements in relation to 'Mrs Manstey's View' (see Chapter 5) which stay outside or above, rather than working emotionally from 'inside', the protagonist's experience (*Eve: Ah, poor woman. She's living life through everyone else. That's to do with her age and her disability. But it's not a life is it. It's restrictive, I think. Fay: You mean it's just – an existence.*) The members of the group, at such times, prefer to be dominated by the compelling force of the group culture rather than to confront their emotional experience and learn or grow from it. What is dreaded 'is the loss of one's sense of security associated with mental change . . . the devastating upheaval of the old order of things . . . the pain of [the] emotional consequences'.[9]

This is serious not only for the reason that, as we saw in Chapter 4, 'a sense of reality matters to the individual in the way that food, drink, air . . . matter'.[10] It is serious, and this is of particular relevance to Shared Reading, because 'the group is essential to the fulfilment of mental life'. 'No real idea can be obtained outside a group itself.'[11] For Bion, 'we are group-ish beings' and 'those elements are operative in us all the time' but only become 'observable when human beings are in visible and audible relation with one another'.[12] We are 'constantly affected', are 'consciously or unconsciously swayed', by our idea of a group and 'this kind of assessment is as much a part of the mental life of the individual as is [the] assessment . . . of the information brought [by the] sense of touch'.[13] Our 'individual psychic make-up' is thus 'intimately related to others'[14] because, as we saw in Chapter 4, our very need to think is generated intersubjectively. The apparatus of thought develops as a means to tolerate, contain and use, rather than suffer from, the 'proto-mental'[15] material, as Bion calls it in *Experiences in Groups* – the most primitive fears, the most basic unformulated experience (that he was later to call 'beta elements'[16]) – first encountered in the primal scene.[17] These elements are thus most susceptible to being mobilized when our 'groupish-ness' is actualized, and it is these 'fearful orientations to reality' which constitute the shared unconscious beliefs of a group and 'shape group experience so profoundly'.[18] 'The group approximates too closely in the minds of the individuals composing it, to the very primitive phantasies about the contents of the mother's body.'[19] It is this 'catastrophic anxiety that occurs at moments of psychic change' that basic assumption mentality 'vigorously defend[s] against'.[20] It is born of 'the group's hatred of having to learn by experience', 'hatred of a process of development' and of the group's wish to be able, 'without undergoing the pains of growth', 'to know exactly how to live and move'.[21] The paradox is this. The group is needed to think at all (as, equivalently, in the small group of the psychoanalytic dyad, 'it requires two minds to come to terms with thoughts derived from one's disturbing emotional experience'[22]). All the while, the group is used to deny or evade thought. 'The power of the group to fulfil the needs of the individual is . . . challenged by the group mentality . . . [the] greatest obstacle to the fulfilment of the aims they wish to achieve by membership of the group.'[23]

The key Bion idea that thinking happens and matures intersubjectively is of critical importance to the therapeutic power of reading, as I described it at the close of Chapter 8. The notion that thinking can also be decisively *blocked* as part of the intersubjective process relates more specifically to the group situation of Shared Reading, and especially to the role of the group leader. The group leader's task, as we shall see more fully in the second part of this chapter, is to encourage a work group mentality by making consistent probing connections with the literary text,[24] directing conversation to it, often to a specific word, line or idea, in order to reconnect the group with the literary text's emotional reality as the ground and stimulus out of which genuine thinking can happen. This focus on the literary work means dispensing with conventional equality and foregoing the idea of putting (what Bion calls) 'good friendly relations' or 'tolerance for differences of opinion' before the deeper needs of the group members, as the leader of the chronic pain reading group acknowledged.

I have to guard against the idea that everybody must 'have their say'. I have to bring people into the conversation of course. But I have to trust the book or the poem to do that. That's why I always try to make sure that the book's presence is felt more than anything else. That way, even if somebody does not speak often, there's still the possibility that they will be reached.

I have to trust the book. A further central tenet of *Experiences in Groups* resonates strongly with this idea of intuitive trust and, indeed, with the findings reported across Part II. For Bion, that is to say, the *test* of the depth of thinking work in the group is 'not [the] words used, but the emotions accompanying them'. This is why Bion reiterates that 'no real idea of [an emotional situation] can be obtained outside [the] group itself'.[25] Intuition is foundational for Bion, as Hinshelwood explains: 'He took as his primary data the experience he himself had while in a working situation . . . [and] picked up these implicit reactions through his sensitivity (intuition) to the emotional atmosphere and how he felt it impelling him to contribute something specific.' It is precisely this 'sensed emotional accompaniment'[26] which guides the group leader in Shared Reading, as we shall see in a moment. The reader will recall, moreover (as I recognized only retrospectively), that it was a kindred type of (consensus) intuition which the research team put to use in analysing the Shared Reading video-recordings – as a means, that is, to distinguish 'hot/live' reading instances (the work group mentality as we may now call it) from 'cold/dead' ones (the defensive basic assumption mentality). As with the group experiences which Bion absorbed and interpreted, these intuited happenings often occurred outside verbal language. Thus, it is to this strata of Shared Reading that I now turn in order to understand and demonstrate, using one representative instance, how work group mode can evolve in Shared Reading.

Becoming a work group in Shared Reading

While non-verbal responses and interactions have by no means been neglected in prior studies of shared reading,[27] I was first alerted to the need for a more systematic analysis of non-verbal features of communication by the linguistic evidence emerging from the transcripts of the chronic pain study. This concluded that there was more construction of 'in-groupness'[28] (through agreement, repetitions and collaborative overlaps) in CBT compared to Shared Reading, where there was found to be little agreement or collaborative overlap between participants. In part, this finding was accounted for by the greater diversity and heterogeneity of language generated by Shared Reading as compared with CBT. Rigorous linguistic analysis of a selection of the transcribed material revealed a relative absence of clinical terms ('nerve blockers') or demotic language ('throbbing') and a tendency towards less conventional use of metaphor ('cocooned in pain').[29] We have seen repeated examples of the literary text stimulating non-standard and personalized syntax and vocabulary in the foregoing chapters. As the consultants put it: in Shared Reading *they're all coming at things from a different angle. The thought processes aren't identical, the language isn't identical. They're saying different things and thinking different things. They have individual impressions and they're finding their own way.* In CBT, by contrast, as the consultants acknowledged, the approach is more didactic. One group member (Holly) unwittingly accounted for the stronger in-group 'we-ness' language among participants in CBT, when she said: *The consultants were very very supportive. But it was the medical professionals there, and the patients here. Try as best we could, it was still a 'them and us' scenario. Whereas in the reading group we are all equal.* The equality was by no means of a merely formal kind to judge by the testimony of group members: *We're not a group, we're a little team you know; A bit like we are brothers and sisters maybe; I feel like I am part of a little family; We're a little community, a little serious community; It's quite telepathic really.* The closeness generated by Shared Reading apparently developed at a level more implicit and profound than the verbalized surface, or at least 'beneath the explicit linguistic markers of co-operative in-groupness'.[30] In what follows, I detail the first steps in an experimental method seeking to capture or understand something of this process.

This work is inspired by the school of empirical microanalysis of mother-infant face-to-face communication, which grew up in the last quarter of the twentieth century, propelled by the now acknowledged pioneers in the field: Daniel Stern, Beatrice Beebe, Ed Tronick, Colwyn Trevarthen, among others. Collectively, these thinkers' research work has demonstrated mother-infant interaction to be a dynamic process of reciprocal, mutually influencing adjustment – or 'attunement' – which organizes a child's experience and emergent sense of self from the beginning: 'From birth, infants live in a two-person social world.' The infant mentally constructs a subjective world of their experience of self and others. 'What is inside', the child's internal life, 'comprises interactive experiences . . . repeated, relatively small [patterns of] self in interaction with another'. Stern calls these 'ways of being with'. Central to these interactive experiences are 'vitality affects', 'kinetic qualities of feeling . . . that correspond to the momentary changes in feeling states involved in the organic processes of being alive' and which are 'experienced as dynamic shifts within ourselves and others'. The world experienced by the infant is primarily 'one of vitality affects before it is a world of formal acts'. 'Affect attunement is so embedded in behaviours, . . . so common and most often so subtle that unless one is looking for it, the attunements will pass unnoticed.' Nonetheless, Stern isolates three general features. Intensity (e.g. the mother's loud voice attunes to the force of the infant's abrupt arm movement during play, vocal matching physical effort); timing (the mother nods her head in time with the infant's shaking of a rattle, matching rhythmic beat and duration); and shape (the mother's head motion or changing vocal pitch borrows the shape of the infant's up and down arm motion). Attunement depends not on mere imitation but on 'behaviours that express the quality of feeling a shared affect state . . . of communing with':

> Tracking and attuning with vitality affects permit one human to 'be with' another in the sense of sharing likely inner experiences on an almost continuous basis. Experience of feeling-connectedness, of being in attunement with one another . . . feels like an unbroken line. It seeks out the activation contour that is momentarily going on in any and every behaviour and uses that contour to keep the thread of communion unbroken.[31]

These attunement behaviours – the occurrence of facial, gestural and vocal modes of expression within a mutually regulated rhythm of pause, reaction time, turn-taking and interruption[32] – were traced using video microanalysis. Beatrice Beebe describes this method (which she learnt to 'love' via Stern's work) as a 'powerful research tool', which taught her to 'see' the 'intricate process of mother-infant moment-to-moment communication'.

> Mother-infant communicative events occur in less than a second. They are so rapid and subtle that they are not quite grasped in real time. By slowing down the movements [slight shifts of gaze, head-up or mouth opening], frame-by-frame, microanalysis identifies beautiful moments [sunbursts of smiles] and disturbing ones [anger, disgust, distress, alarm] and [illustrates how] relatively small amounts of nonverbal communication carry enormous information.

'This visual grounding', says Beebe, 'gave the work a visceral, intuitive, and immediate form of comprehension'. It enabled a fine-grained and 'potent assessment of the emotional quality of the relationship',[33] capable, across multiple mother-infant dyads, of specifying communication processes at four months which predicted attachment outcomes at twelve months. Significantly, secure attachment depended not on high coordination of communicative behaviours, which was deemed over-vigilant monitoring on the part of the parent (as low coordination bespoke withdrawal). Rather, optimal coordination was 'midrange' leaving 'more "space", more room for uncertainty, initiative and flexibility within the experience of correspondence and contingency',[34] as well as richer experience, on a continuum of engagement and disengagement, of 'forms of being with'.

A key element of Beebe's research, one which first drew me to this field, has been concerned with using the insights gained from her mother-infant research to better understand how they are foundational for adult psychopathology and interpersonal relations, and to inform her therapeutic practice with adults. Both aspects are relevant to the dynamics of literary reading groups, as we shall see later in this chapter and the next. Indeed, findings from this collaborative school of work have already been applied (albeit sparingly thus far) to therapeutic arts activities, such as dance.[35]

This book has so far been concerned principally with elucidating the vitality affects produced by the *literary work*. When we asked, as a research team, 'Is this instance "alive" or not?', often, as I have begun to indicate in previous chapters, the vitality signal was (or was accompanied by) a non-verbal one, especially when (as we saw with Michael) the reader is lost for words. But often the moments we have scrutinized have also catalysed a vitality affect within the group. It is this vital 'interpersonality'[36] between the individual, the literary text and the group, and its effect on the experience of a community, that we have sought to locate using our own version of microanalysis of the video-recordings of the reading sessions. This has inevitably proved to be a compromised endeavour. While the recordings lend themselves in some ways to the ethological approach favoured by Stern (which privileges 'the careful description of behaviour in its natural habitat, detailing the form, sequence and timing of behaviour'[37]), they were not purpose-made for this undertaking. Microanalysis of caregivers and infants involves dyads exclusively and makes use of two cameras, one for each partner, for split-screen analysis of interaction. The reading group was made up of anything between three and ten people interacting, sometimes many of them at once, who were filmed by a single camera. Thus, early into this endeavour, we were aware that we would have to limit ourselves to isolation of features that could be used to design future scientific studies set up for this purpose, using multiple cameras. Despite these limitations, our findings have been arresting both at a local level and in terms of their cumulative impact across the reading sessions and, as we shall see, have tended to confirm the group leader and participants' sense that certain sessions were defining in 'knitting' the group together.

What follows is a representative example, divided into three short movements, of the kind of vitality affects we identified. These are signalled in the transcript extracts by the abbreviation VA, sequentially numbered. This is a loose and intuitive, rather than scientific or comprehensive, notation system and is principally designed to enable ease of reference in the ensuing discussion.

The session in question took place towards the end of the study (in Week 20). It is unusually close to the end of the allocated time when the group begins to look at W. B. Yeats's 'The Lake Isle of Innisfree'. As always happens, the group leader reads aloud, while the group members silently read the text in front of them.

> I will arise and go now, and go to Innisfree,
> And a small cabin build there, of clay and wattles made;
> Nine bean-rows will I have there, a hive for the honey-bee,
> And live alone in the bee-loud glade.
>
> And I shall have some peace there, for peace comes dropping slow,
> Dropping from the veils of the morning to where the cricket sings;
> There midnight's all a glimmer, and noon a purple glow,
> And evening full of the linnet's wings.
>
> I will arise and go now, for always night and day
> I hear lake water lapping with low sounds by the shore;
> While I stand on the roadway, or on the pavements grey,
> I hear it in the deep heart's core.[38]

Movement one

At the completion of the final line, John, his eyes on the page in front of him, nods firmly, chin and bottom lip pushed out in an expression of strong assent. (VA1) Otherwise, the group members continue to look silently at the poem, taking it in. The group leader suggests reading the poem again, asking whether anyone would like to take a turn reading. Deborah says (quietly), *I will.* Susan then offers to share the reading: *We could have one piece each.* Susan is self-conscious about her reading ability (she has a diagnosis of dyslexia) and has shown reluctance to read aloud in previous sessions. Volunteering to do so is new for her. Her reading of the first stanza is quite faltering and fragmented. Deborah (who is an animated speaker) reads the second stanza at an unusually slow (albeit rhythmic) pace. Mary, reading from the page with everyone else, glances up at Deborah as she begins to read the second line and does so again at the close of lines three and four. (VA2) Susan's reading of the third stanza is markedly more fluent, borrowing tempo and rhythm from Deborah's reading. (VA3) At 'always night and day', Mary begins (just audibly, only Eve visibly notices), eyes now firmly on the poem, to read along with Susan. (VA4) At the final line, John once again nods, gently this time and several times, saying 'Mmm' affirmatively. (VA5)

Group Leader: It's says 'I will arise and go now'. What do you think . . .? Is he even – really going to go or . . .?

Deborah [who has been staring thoughtfully into the distance while everyone is looking down at the poem]: I don't know whether he is physically going or . . .?

Susan: No, I don't think he's physically going. I think it's an internal thing. Maybe you are so stressed out, maybe you need to put the shutters down and just – sort yourself out. [The gaze of the whole group is now directed towards the speakers. (VA6)]

Group Leader: So an inner thing – yet all these details as well. [She re-reads stanza one].

At line 2, 'A small cabin build there', Mary, who is seated next to the group leader, again begins to read along, more audibly this time. (VA7) The group leader notices this immediately (as do Eve, Holly and Michael in time) and begins to nod rhythmically as she reads, looking frequently towards Mary. (VA8)

Group Leader: [directly as she stops reading stanza one]: Do you like that Mary? Do you like reading it?

Mary: [looking up at the group leader in surprise, as if awoken from a reverie]. Yes, it's nice [quietly].

Group Leader: It sounds lovely doesn't it?

Mary: Yes, it does.

Michael and Deborah both look towards Mary and, unaware of one another's response, instinctively smile during this exchange. (VA9)

*   *   *

Mary, as we saw in Chapter 6, rarely spoke in the group and had never before read aloud, though she had *frequently* told the consultants (as they put it) *how much she gets out of the reading group: she is definitely right in there with it, something is going on for her.* Mary's verbalizing of the words of the poem, as if to herself, on this occasion was one of the few signs she ever gave of 'something going on' inside her.

Mary is attuned to the poem's 'sound', its music, first and foremost. In Shared Reading, both poem and sound are always, initially at least, mediated by the group leader. A key effect of the text's being read aloud, carefully and caringly, is that the poem or story is closer to a 'voiced embodied presence' than a two-dimensional text.[39] As participants in the chronic pain group variously expressed it: *Things become more 3D and more alive; It is just cold words on the page until it is read aloud; It doesn't have any passion, or really any meaning. It often looks indecipherable; I've never read poetry before. I've connected with the poetry because it is read aloud. It seems to – resonate; It makes a difference, the voiceover. It creates a stillness and peace in the room.* The group leader's task is to sustain the atmosphere first created by the poem. What in fact happens in the few minutes described in slow motion above is that the vitality affect of reading aloud is first transmitted by the group leader to group members who then keep the transmission affect alive through their own reading aloud. This is most apparent in Mary's strikingly involuntary and unusual verbal responsiveness. But it is visibly felt across the group, in clear instances of Stern's broad categories of affect attunement. VA3 to VA5 and VA7 are prominent examples of attuned timing, between Deborah and Susan, Susan and Mary, and Mary and the group leader, which is simultaneous with, and catalysed by, the rhythm of the poem. The group leader's nodding to the beat and duration of Mary's reading (VA8) is an example of attuned timing and shape at once, and, like John's nods (VA1 and VA5), both matches the intensity of the emotional resonance of the poem's final lines, and, at the same time, their affect as they are read aloud here and now in the room. 'Adult face-to-face communication', says Beatrice Beebe, 'is very similar to mother-infant communication'. The non-verbal behaviours which are highly influential – 'gaze shifts, slight changes in facial expression or head orientation' – are 'almost imperceptible' and 'largely nonconscious, out of awareness'. This 'implicit'[40] form of processing seems to be at work in the attunements which are out of conscious awareness in this extract: the mutual gaze shift at VA6 and the involuntarily matching smiles at VA9. The intersubjective emotional resonance that is thus transmitted and registered subvocally and subconsciously now serves to densen the felt seriousness of the discussion. The session has already begun to run over its allotted time, but everyone is intently present.

Movement two

Group Leader:Is it real . . .? Have they been here or – Is it a real place?
Eve: Is it somewhere he's left?
Mary: [reading and pointing to the line] 'I shall have some peace there'. (VA10)
*Holly: Or somewhere he hasn't been to yet. He's saying 'I **will** arise and go now'.*
*Deborah: It's right here in the present too. 'I will arise and go **now.**'*
John: Is he dreaming it?
Susan: It's your inner dreams, isn't it? [animatedly, her whole hand clutching toward her heart at 'inner']. (VA11) It's the things that you wish you can do, just wish you could go there now and everyone – leave me alone.

Eve: A space they imagine they've got.
Deborah [who has again been looking ahead intently throughout these
*   exchanges]:Like an inner freedom.*
Mary [once more reading and pointing to the line]:Where's he's saying, 'I
*   shall have some peace there'. (VA12)*

The group leader now joins in with Mary in re-reading the middle stanza, leaving Mary to re-read the last two lines solo, and nodding to the rhythm once more.

Mary [after a long pause]: I like the last verse. [She re-reads the final
*   stanza again, in full, on her own.] The sound of the shore, water lapping*
*   on the shore [using her hands to express a gentle flowing movement],*
*   I think that's lovely. (VA13)*
Deborah: Sort of soothing. Shhh, shhh, constantly [mimicking Mary's own
*   hand movements to express the lapping water]. (VA14) Restful. And*
*   it does drop on, doesn't it, when you relax, from your head down your*
*   body [drawing the movement with her hands]. Stress builds up [hands*
*   move up body strugglingly, face tightens], but peace*
Deborah, Group leader, Susan, Mary [in unison]: Drops down. (VA15)

What is striking about this sequence is that, as other group members probe the 'space' of the poem – where it is, even *whether* it is – Mary is already inhabiting it (VA10, VA12, VA13) and has been doing so virtually from the start of the session. At VA14 and VA15, first Deborah, then Susan and the group leader (verbally), and then the whole group (implicitly), join her there. Their arrival is signalled by their predicting and completing – and vocally and tonally expressing (in a falling cadence on 'down') – what Deborah begins: a rhythmic-semantic sense unit which has the force of a poetic epigram ('Stress builds up, peace drops down'). At every level, this is a palpable moment of group synchrony, of those present inhabiting 'one mind time and one body related space' as Colwyn Trevarthen describes the intimate intersubjective coordination between caregiver and infant.[41]

Movement three

Michael, who is seated on the other side of the group leader, and has been leaning back for the whole session, begins to lean forward in the last movement, better to see and hear Joan. (V16)

Michael: I still can't figure this part at the end, 'I will arise and go now, for
*   always night and day'. [His appeal is directly to the group leader, but*

> *the question cues every group member to return to look at the text as one. (VA17)] Is this a person content now, sort of at rest?*
> *Group Leader: Yes, it's the same line twice over, isn't it? 'I will arise and go now, and go to Innisfree', 'I will arise and go now, for always . . .'*
> *Holly: I don't think – I don't think it means go there forever. I think it means. . . 'for always night and day' he hears the lake water.*
> *Mary [reading the lines of the final stanza aloud – to herself, but audibly to all (VA18)]: 'While I stand on the roadway, or on the pavements grey,/I hear it in the deep heart's core.'*
> *Deborah: While he is standing on a busy street, he can hear the shore moving instead. Getting away from the here and now.*
> *Michael: The sounds just fade away, everything else is kind of gone. You've just got your thoughts, you're left with only those, nothing else. You've gone deep into yourself.*
> *Deborah: Deep into the heart's core. [John and Holly nod: everyone is looking up and towards Michael now. (VA19)]*
> *Holly: It can be – anything, any situation you find yourself in.*
> *Michael: It doesn't matter where you are. . . your peace is inside. [Knocks at his heart. (VA20)]*

That final action (VA20) mirrors Susan's earlier emphatic motioning towards her heart (V11) – an out of awareness signal of one space, one mind, catalysed by the poem's own deep centre, 'the heart's core'. When the consultant viewed this session, he was 'fascinated' by the way the dialogue, wherein the group members are so in tune with one another, is at the same time *almost in the same rhythm as the poem: their minds are operating along with the movement of the poem*. What he meant by this was that the conversation kept returning to the idea of something 'inner', some internal space or peace or freedom; and, as in the poem, each new wave ('I will arise and go') was not 'to' somewhere, but rather a movement deeper or closer 'inside'. In this regard, Deborah's unaccustomed staring into the distance in Movements One and Two was a kind of mirroring analogue, or an alternative sense-mode, for Mary's repeated return to the sound of the poem.

In many ways, the (albeit limited) slow-motion viewing of interaction between person, poem and others simply verifies what we intuited early in our study of Shared Reading. That is to say, the group does 'not really exist save as a static or notional unit until, through the text and the group leader serving it, live connections are made between one individual and another. Then its movements, connections and reconfigurations between different individuals at different moments in relation to different texts are unpredictable'.[42] As one person, now another, becomes the 'realizer' of the text or of a personal meaning, the centre suddenly shifts or a new alignment occurs in a dynamic process of fluid and spontaneous grouping and regrouping. We have seen this phenomenon throughout Part II, in fact. Think of David in relation to 'The Liar' or Susan and Deborah responding to 'Mysteriously Standing' – all temporarily hold or embody the text's emotional 'inside'. There was a strong sense from the group leader (and more implicitly from group members who involuntarily recalled and referenced the session in later ones) that the reading of 'Mrs Manstey's View' was a turning point in the group's history, a defining session in turning it from a gathering of individuals into a 'serious community', because the holding of the story's emotional meaning was richly and multiply shared. A crude, non-analytical count of vitality affects in that session shows a decided increase in relation to previous sessions (though this cannot be taken as a mathematically accurate guide given that the group size continuously altered). More reliably indicative than the evidence of any single session is the number of VAs involving individual group members. Michael, for example, was very quiet and habitually passive in the early sessions. This was the Michael the consultants were accustomed to, a person who was *self-effacing and managed to blend into the background*: indeed, on first observing the video footage of the early sessions of the group, Michael seemed almost invisible to them (*I kept thinking 'where is he?'* said one consultant). Michael's verbal contributions and vital non-verbal attunements increased markedly (and more than any other group member's) across the study, spiking in certain sessions, 'The Visitor' session included. Indeed, the reader may recall that Michael's emphatic non-verbal action in that session (the boldest he ever performed) of extending his arm forwards across the table in imitation of a clock hand (when saying that as a child *he used to try to will the hand to stop*) was itself an instance of attuned shaping, copying Fay's use of her own hand a moment before to trace in the air the movement of the clock's hand. It is worth remarking also that the group leader's question in response – *Why, was that because of something you didn't want to happen?* – was itself a vitality affect, emerging naturalistically and spontaneously out of the instant's mutual attentiveness, neither predicting nor seeking the powerful effect it produced. The group leader is at one level analogous to, or a type of, the ideal co-creating analyst we witnessed in the previous chapter, intuiting the next move or word, not in order to target painful memory, but so as to deepen inner probing. 'Spontaneity has more value for the patient than a conventional pseudo-tolerant discourse which will be experienced by the patient as artificial and governed by technical manuals.'[43] In fact, the group leader's role, moment by moment, is always determined by the dynamic intersubjectivities and affects produced, first and foremost, by the literary text. It is not uncommon for the group leader to cede her role of centring or enabling meaning-making entirely to a group participant. Think of Eve 'diagnosing' the cause of Holly's pain. Or of Holly herself holding the mental-emotional terrain of Elizabeth Jennings's lines on recognitions 'missed' or 'not guessed'. It is the cumulative increase of such vitality affects, across group members and the group leader, rather than individual defining moments, that powers the *bond of intimacy* which the group leader herself described as *almost cellular. Perhaps it has to do*, she suggested, *with the implicit shared experience of suffering, living and thinking with pain, which is curious insofar as group members rarely talk about their pain directly. It is as though the story or poem acts as a carrier for our shared pain, holding us together as one body, one mind.*

What is remarkable about the reading instance discussed above is that the key vitality affect, the one that drives the gravitational pull, comes from and happens entirely within the language and music of the text. In total, Mary re-read the words of the poem (aloud or almost) five times, and used few words besides those of the poem. Out of the awareness of Mary herself, this was sufficient to catalyse the coalescence of the group members around it. As Mary herself put it in the interview, witnessing the footage.

Oh yes I remember that. I did love it yes. But I didn't know I was reading it with her you know. I shouldn't have been doing that. I just love that poem – that part. I couldn't resist reading it myself. It really got into me. And everybody seemed to get carried away with it.

Mary gave no indication that she had encountered the poem before. But, of all the group members, she was the only one of the generation who might have experienced poetry recitation at school. As Catherine Robson puts it in *Heart Beats: Everyday Life and the Memorized Poem)*, 'a poem committed to heart in childhood could bring much-needed solace to an adult in psychological pain'.[44] It is possible that something of the remembered power of vocalized poetry was working in Mary at this moment.

But what Robson calls the 'emotional history'[45] of voiced poetry is older and deeper still. In a rigorous analysis of baby-talk or motherese – the verbal language that accompanies and is inseparable from the close temporal coordination of actions and responses between mother and infant – David Miall and Ellen Dissanayake found this language to possess dynamic poetic features and textures: rhythmic repetition; regular stress and accent; interspersed pauses and rests; distinct pitch contours; and a varying range of tempo, emphasis, vigour and amplitude (loud/soft, fast/slow). In its hyperbole, parallelism, exaggerated undulation of vocal shapes and generally high degree of patterned or structural repetition (rhyme, rhythm), mother-infant sing-song is, Miall and Dissanayake propose, 'an elementary form of foregrounding . . . preliminary to its more developed form in poetry'.[46] Such prosodic (metrical and phonetic) features, that is to say, reveal a rudimentary poetics, the 'affective, prelinguistic and pre-literate substrates' of poetry, which 'have deep roots in our ancestral and individual non-verbal past [and] are affecting because of their biological importance'. Babies display 'innate receptiveness to fundamental proto-aesthetic devices that evolved to enable these earliest adult/infant interactions'.[47] Verbal interaction between caregiver and infant (which of course has no lexical meaning for the latter) is thus 'primarily a resource for effects at the level of sound – i.e. the intonation, rhythm and phonetic colour afforded by the words'[48] – to stimulate emotional coordination and attuned affective interaction. For an infant, that is to say, the meaning of a mother's speech is *'purely* [its] paralinguistic affinitive messages'.[49] This means that 'although baby talk, like poetry, defamiliarizes verbal language, at least from the adult's perspective, to the baby it is presumably familiar and natural. To the baby, it is the "poetry", not the everyday language that is the norm'.[50]

It is as if, then, Mary becomes the heartbeat of the group, and the group members beat with her, so to speak, because as humans, they are biologically primed to do so. On the one hand, this preliterate affective 'training' in foregrounded language accounts, in Miall's and Dissanayake's thesis, for the adult receptivity to its occurrences in literature, which we have witnessed across Part II. On the other hand, it also helps explain how the poetic in literature as a discourse can provide ready access to the primitive pre-verbal world, not capable of expression in words, which Melanie Klein called 'memories in feelings',[51] and from which fundamental insight Bion's theories of groups and thinking came largely to depend.[52] Critically, perhaps, it is *Shared* Reading, as we have just now seen, which has the power thus to release vital affective resources not only analogous to, but first learnt between, caregiver and infant. 'This innate rhythmic musicality', 'the distant past still present in live speech', provides, says Trevarthen, 'the prosodic background for all lyrical urges to communicate affectively'.[53] The re-creation through stories and poems of the 'intimacy of a shared verbal space'[54] in Shared Reading arguably recovers and helps fulfil an often lost or neglected need for such 'emotional communion' – an idea to which I return in Part III.

Reading not talking

Pain, trauma, treatment

10

Pain and stuckness

Parts I and II have emphasized the relationship between literary reading and psychoanalysis, firstly, because of the historical and continuing affinity between literature and psychoanalytic theory and practice; and, secondly, because the influential psychologies of reading to which I have been indebted in Chapter 2 have had recourse (as have I) to psychoanalytic thought in explicating reading processes. What I venture in this chapter is that, in terms of its therapeutic potential, literary reading (shared or otherwise) lies somewhere between traditional psychoanalysis and psychosocial interventions, which are increasingly in use in relation to chronic pain as an alternative to CBT, the 'gold standard' intervention. My intention is to emphasize literary reading's practical value as a therapeutic aid that can be mobilized in relation to a range of therapies recognized in chronic pain care. In so doing, I call upon for the first time – and indeed in this chapter predominantly – relevant recent work in neuroscience which, sometimes explicitly, is seeking to rescue the value of literature for modern life.[1]

'Psychological flexibility'

Psychosocial interventions in chronic pain are increasingly informed and framed by the concept of 'psychological flexibility'. The term refers to the 'ability to be fully present in the current moment, and from that position, to be able to either maintain or to change one's behaviour to more successfully pursue that which is most personally important, according to what the situation directly affords'.[2] The model emphasizes, on the one hand, direct and open awareness of emotions, sensations and thoughts, including unwanted ones, without being restricted by, or attempting to control, them; and, on the other hand, acting on the basis of long-term values and beliefs rather than on short-term reactive impulses or unhelpful response-narrowing thoughts. 'This way of behaving', say those advocating the use of the concept of psychological flexibility in chronic pain care, 'can be contrasted to directing one's efforts toward the suppression of unwanted thoughts, avoidance of uncomfortable feelings or sensations, distraction away from current experience, or attempts to alter pain intensity, particularly when these responses interfere with goal attainment and values pursuit over the longer term'.[3] Thus, the rationale for encouraging psychological flexibility is that for people living with chronic pain 'a primary source of suffering [is] psychological *in*flexibility' (my emphasis) which occurs when cognitive processes, such as learning from instructions or rules, or engaging in problem-solving or reasoning, 'overwhelm' the effects of other behavioural processes. 'Avoidant behaviour can be rigid, and fail to change even with the evidence of its clearly disabling effects; or otherwise healthy behaviour can be non-persistent, stopping whenever pain or a worry occurs. In either case, the behaviour patterns seem likely to result in significantly reduced functioning in the long term.'[4]

Over the past two decades, the therapy most associated with psychological flexibility, Acceptance and Commitment Therapy (ACT), has been increasingly recognized as an intervention in relation to chronic pain. The 'acceptance' element of ACT focuses on increased willingness to *have* pain, to experience its discomfort without struggle or unhelpful efforts to control or avoid it. This involves emphasis on awareness of emotional conflict and purposeful acknowledgement of troubling mental events in order to alter the 'stimulus function of pain such that it no longer unavoidably occasions disability behaviour'.[5] ACT's 'commitment' element fosters 'a present-focused ability to identify persistent and problematic pain avoidance strategies and shift those efforts toward pursuing values and living a meaningful life'. Committed action, that is to say, 'takes place in the "here and now", and is part of an actively chosen path taken in the service of underlying values'.[6] ACT-based interventions have shown benefits in terms of: pain-related distress, depression and anxiety; frequency of pain-related health visits; current work status; physical functioning; emotional functioning; and physical task persistence. There is also promising evidence of the longer-term impact of increased engagement in valued activity beyond treatment, a key consideration in relation to chronic pain, where the obstinacy of symptoms requires 'consistent engagement in new patterns of behaviour . . . that may be in some ways unnatural given the persistence of pain'.[7]

In many ways, ACT is an extension and evolution of CBT insofar as it targets responses to pain rather than pain itself, in order that altered responses lead to decreased disability. But ACT represents a clear shift away from emphasizing coping and pain management strategies. In part, this is because the efficacy of such methods has been difficult to establish, and there is evidence to suggest that CBT's power to alleviate suffering owes more to the psychological flexibility it indirectly encourages rather than the adaptive behaviours it directly seeks to inculcate.[8] But ACT also seeks, through its orientation towards present fluid awareness of sensation, to reduce dependence on verbal problem-solving and the ways that actions and behaviours are 'caught up'[9] with inflexible language and cognitive patterns. In this respect, ACT's closer affinity is with mindfulness, defined by Jon Kabat-Zinn (who first introduced the Eastern practice of meditation into Western healthcare, specifically, in the first instance, as a treatment for chronic pain) as 'the awareness that emerges through paying attention on purpose, in the present moment, and nonjudgmentally to the unfolding of experience moment by moment'.[10] Kabat-Zinn's development of Mindfulness-Based Stress Reduction (MBSR) – an eight-week programme of intensive training in meditation and its practice and application for daily living – led to a series of studies in the 1980s on the impact of MBSR for people living with chronic pain. These found significant changes in self-reported experience of pain intensity, and in mood, energy for daily activity, anxiety and depression, independent of the nature of their pain condition, with evidence of prolonged effect over years.[11] The detached observation of pain sensation, as well as of internal mental states (thoughts, emotions, impulses and memories), appears, according to Kabat-Zinn, to 'cause an "uncoupling" of the sensory dimension of the pain experience from the affective/evaluative alarm reaction' and 'reduce the experience of suffering via cognitive reappraisal'.[12] The use of mindfulness-based interventions as part of integrated, multidisciplinary pain management plans has been increasingly endorsed by research which broadly replicates Kabat-Zinn's findings (albeit with more modest evidence of success).[13] Mindfulness has been found to alleviate psychological symptoms and behaviours (catastrophizing, fear avoidance, pain hypervigilance) which (as we saw in Chapter 1) amplify pain experience and contribute to functional disability.[14] In addition, brain imaging studies over the last two decades have indicated that central nervous system pain perception pathways may be inhibited or regulated through mindfulness.[15] These studies have supported Kabat-Zinn's theory of the uncoupling of pain and affect by indicating that both sensory and affective aspects of the perception of pain may be modulated through the self-regulation of attention that is inculcated through the practice of mindfulness.[16] Mindfulness has been shown to increase the activation of brain regions implicated in cognitive and emotional control during anticipation of pain, and this neural activity is associated with reduced experience of pain unpleasantness.[17] One hypothesis is that, in focusing mental awareness on the present moment, away from either past or future experience, meditation alters the emotional appraisal of pain by withdrawing attention from anticipation of unpleasantness and/or by cultivating an attitude of acceptance towards impending stimuli.[18] Such findings resonate with the experience of participants of Shared Reading, for whom reading *removed the pain to a different place*. 'It was as though the extra mental effort helped shift immersion to another level and blocked out the pain more successfully.'[19] These brain imaging studies may throw light by analogy, therefore, on the neural processes by which participants experienced relief from pain symptoms both during and after reading sessions.

Indeed, it is difficult *not* to draw together the affinities between the practices and effects of Shared Reading, ACT and MBSR. Though one focuses on a literary text, one on personal values and one on daily meditative practice, all concentrate on the here and now and on being 'open', 'aware' and psychologically 'active' in relation to present experience.[20] None directly target the minimizing of pain. Rather, they work (intentionally or otherwise) by 'changing the relationship with pain'.[21] All three challenge the goal-driven emphasis of CBT – on 'identifying thoughts as distorted and in need of change'[22] and prescribing alteration in behavioural responses – by focusing on increased contact, and often confrontation, with (difficult) experience rather than wishing it away. 'Psychological flexibility' might be posited as the process which underlies and unites all three practices and accounts for benefits which accrue from them in respect of the subjective-emotional experience of pain.

'Bottom-up therapy'

At another level, however, Shared Reading's alignment with practices which emphasize embodiment is utterly surprising. For Shared Reading does not (any more than the literary text upon which it is based) eschew thought and cognition. Rather, as Part II will have made clear, it embraces and encourages the release of emotion into conscious articulate comprehension. As such, Shared Reading might readily be categorized as one of the species of 'talk' therapy, which proponents of therapies emphasizing awareness of the present moment and the embodied mind regard with suspicion. It is likely that Bessel van der Kolk, for example, the psychiatrist who 'discovered' PTSD when he was working at the US Veterans Association, would be the first to baulk at the idea that talking – and talking about books of all things! – could intervene in lives riven by pain. 'For a hundred years or more, every textbook of psychology and psychotherapy has advised that some method of talking about distressing feelings can resolve them. However, I am continually impressed by how difficult it is for people who have gone through the unspeakable to convey the essence of their experience.'[23] Van der Kolk's field is trauma, principally in relation to veterans and survivors of child abuse – experiences and groups which, as we have seen, are especially vulnerable to developing chronic pain.

Van der Kolk frequently acknowledges the association in his acclaimed and influential, if controversial,[24] book, *The Body Keeps the Score,* in which he makes a neurological and psychiatric case for favouring 'bottom-up' therapies that put people in 'visceral' contact with trauma over both pharmacological interventions and those that operate 'top-down – by talking'. His reasoning, based on extensive clinical evidence, is that talk therapies begin too 'high up' in cognitive functioning. 'While we all want to move beyond trauma, the part of our brain that is devoted to ensuring survival (deep down below our rational brain) is not very good at denial. Long after a traumatic event is over, it may be reactivated at the slightest hint of danger and mobilise disturbed brain circuits and massive amounts of stress hormones.'[25] The 'emotional brain' to which van der Kolk here refers is said to be composed of the evolutionarily older brain structures which are the first to be activated by sensory input posing a threat – what neuroscientist Joseph LeDoux calls the 'quick and dirty' neural pathway (or 'low road') to triggering responses in relation to dangerous stimuli. The latter's quick transmission bypasses the 'high road',[26] van der Kolk's 'rational brain' or the processing systems believed to be involved in thinking, reasoning and consciousness (such as the PFC discussed in Chapter 1), and essential to overriding the emergency response. If the threat is experienced as too intense or the higher brain system's filter system is too weak, as is typical in trauma survivors, there is nothing to control the automatic response. A state of high alert and sensory overload results. Brain activity is rekindled as if the trauma were actually occurring, unmodified by the passage of time. Triggers can occur in multiple aspects of daily experience, precipitating intense emotions, physical sensations and impulsive actions which feel incomprehensible and overwhelming because trauma itself interferes with the awareness that one is re-experiencing and re-enacting the past. 'Emotions and physical sensations imprinted during the trauma are experienced not as memories but as disruptive physical reactions in the present.' It is because 'the past is alive in terms of gnawing interior discomfort', and not impressed upon the mind merely, that traumatized people 'feel chronically unsafe within their bodies'. This hypervigilance and sensitivity in response to threat produces actual physiological changes – akin to physical lesions like strokes – resulting in 'a fundamental reorganisation of the way mind and brain manage perceptions' which directly connects to the development of chronic pain:

> After trauma the world is experienced with a different nervous system. The survivor's energy now becomes focused on suppressing inner chaos, on *not* thinking about what has happened and not feeling residues of terror and panic in their bodies, at the expense of spontaneous involvement in their lives. These attempts to maintain control over unbearable physiological reactions can result in a whole range of physical symptoms, including

fibromyalgia, chronic fatigue, and other autoimmune diseases. This explains why it is critical for trauma treatment to engage the entire organism, body, mind and brain.[27]

Moreover, merely 'telling the story' of what has happened is not enough, since doing so 'doesn't necessarily alter the automatic physical and hormonal responses of bodies that remain hypervigilant, prepared to be assaulted or violated at any time'. Most of van der Kolk's patients were, anyway, unable 'to make their past into a story that happened long ago': 'even years later traumatised people often have enormous difficulty telling other people what has happened to them. [The feelings their bodies re-experience] are almost impossible to articulate. Trauma by nature drives us to the edge of comprehension, cutting us off from language based on common experience or an imaginable past'.[28] One key finding of van der Kolk's clinical work was that during PTSD sufferers' flashbacks, the images of past trauma activated the right hemisphere of the brain (intuitive, emotional, visual, reacting to sound, touch, smell) and deactivated the left (linguistic, analytical, naming things and understanding their interrelationships). The disabling of the left side of the brain 'has a direct impact on the capacity to organise experience into logical sequences and to translate our shifting feelings and perceptions into words' such that people 'may not be aware that they are reexperiencing and reenacting the past'. This does not mean, van der Kolk goes on, that people are wholly unable to talk about a tragedy that has befallen them. On the contrary:

> Sooner or later most survivors . . . come up with what many of them call their 'cover story' that offers some explanation for their symptoms and behaviour for public consumption. These stories, however, rarely capture the inner truth of the experience. . . . It is so much easier to talk about what has been done to them – to tell a story of victimisation and revenge – than to notice, feel, and put into words the reality of their internal experience.

'For real change to take place, the body needs to learn that the danger has passed and to live in the reality of the present.'[29]

High on van der Kolk's list of therapies which enable such learning are those based on meditative practice – mindfulness and yoga in particular. *The Body Keeps the Score* reports extensive studies finding that yoga can help traumatized people 'learn to comfortably inhabit their tortured bodies' through its attention to breathing; rhythms of tension and relaxation in the muscles of the face, trunk and limbs; and sensation, moment to moment. 'These shifts carry the essence of the organism's responses: the emotional states that are imprinted in the body's chemical profile.' Reconnecting with the continual shifts in inner sensory worlds was found to change physiology, including increasing heart rate variability. Heart rate fluctuations are a sign of emotional and physical health which are lacking in people 'shut-down' by trauma, negatively affecting responses to stress and emotion regulation. Learning to tolerate physical sensations for what they are – existing in the present, transient, finite – renders those that are the 'unbidden residue of a terrible past' also temporary and not 'unending threats to life today', leaving a person 'stuck forever in a helpless state of horror'. The costs of not learning to change one's relationship to physical sensation are all too familiar:

> One of the ways the memory of helplessness is stored is as muscle tension or feelings of disintegration in affected body areas (head, back, limbs). Constant muscle tension leads to spasms, back pain, migraine headaches . . . and other forms of chronic pain. [Sufferers] may visit multiple specialists, undergo extensive diagnostic tests, and be prescribed multiple medications, some of which may provide temporary relief but all of which fail to address the underlying issues. Their diagnosis will come to define their reality without ever being defined as a symptom of their attempt to deal with trauma. [Lives] come to revolve around bracing against and neutralising unwanted sensory experiences and becoming experts in self-numbing.[30]

As we saw in Chapter 1, such bracing and self-numbing have their own brain signature in reduced grey matter and connectivity in chronic pain sufferers. Indeed, there is a strong synergy between the neuroscientific evidence van der Kolk cites in relation to yoga and trauma and analogous research concerning pain. Studies have indicated an association between meditative practice and structural changes in areas of the brain critical for sensory, cognitive and emotional processing. Specifically, experienced meditators have been found to exhibit an increase in grey matter concentration in multiple brain regions involved in learning and memory, emotion regulation, self-referential processing and perspective-taking.[31] Investigating the possible neuroanatomical underpinnings of the beneficial effects for pain of yoga specifically (benefits often attributed to yoga's effect on the strength and flexibility of the musculoskeletal system), Villemure et al. also found increased grey matter in multiple cortical regions in yoga practitioners – especially those related to affective pain processing and pain regulation – together with twice the tolerance of pain in yoga practitioners relative to non-practitioners. The authors propose that by teaching cognitive strategies to deal with sensory inputs and the potential emotional reactions attached to these inputs, yoga thereby strengthens connectivity in the brain areas stimulated. As neuroplasticity dictates that the more you use part of the brain, the more useful it becomes, so the more often yoga activates pain awareness centres, the more aware they become. The rule that 'neurons that fire together wire together'[32] is the explanation for the default setting of the chronic pain brain, which we encountered in Chapter 1. The emotional and cognitive tools developed in yoga (focused attention and introspective observation of phenomenal experiences as they are encountered) potentially alter a person's relationship with pain, that is to say, by altering brain anatomy and reversing those defaults.

For van der Kolk, the key value of utilizing the brain's natural neuroplasticity is to help people whose experiences have 'compromised the physical embodied feeling of being alive'. 'Being traumatised is not just an issue of being stuck in the past: it is just as much a problem of not being fully alive in the present.' Unable to integrate experiences into ongoing life, people 'continue to be "there" and do not know how to be "here"'.[33] All the therapeutic methods van der Kolk describes and recommends involve confrontation, therefore, with what has happened, minus the re-traumatization that habitually accompanies it. One of the most successful of these methods is eye movement desensitization and reprocessing (EMDR, recommended for PTSD in the UK National Institute for Health and Care Excellence guidelines). In EMDR, people are supported in recollection of traumatic experiences, while receiving rhythmic stimuli in a left-to-right pattern (such as following with their eyes a finger moving slowly side to side repeatedly). The process frees up emotions, sensations, images and thoughts hitherto frozen, locked-down and embedded in the body, which are then reprocessed, reassembled and reintegrated into continuing life. The reasons for EDMR's effects are not fully understood; in addition to the direct impact on brain regions and physiology (lowered heart rate, slower breathing, decreased skin conductance), one possibility is that the process is related to the dreaming which occurs in Rapid Eye Movement sleep, and that the kind of creative recombination of apparently unrelated fragments of experience which dreams enact enables effective memory processing and trauma resolution. In van der Kolk's accounts of the process, patients first get inside the reality of the memory, its feel, sights, sounds; stay inside aided by the bilateral stimulation, and the therapist's ('Notice this' 'Hold that', 'Take a deep breath') prompts; and emerge from it with the intensity behind them ('It's over . . . has become the story of a terrible event that happened long ago'). The rule is that people have to be supported to experience the intensity in order to be released from it.

Visiting the past in therapy should happen while people are, biologically speaking, firmly rooted in the present and feeling as calm, safe and grounded as possible. ('Grounded' means that you can feel your butt in your chair, see the light coming through the window, feel the tension in your calves, and hear the wind stirring the tree outside.) Being anchored in the present while revisiting the trauma opens the possibility of deeply knowing that the terrible events belong to the past.[34]

In view of this account, I want to venture that Shared Reading might be regarded – and used – as a partially equivalent 'therapy', one which likewise has the capacity to render emotional pain safely present, even while breaching habitual defences, catching readers preconsciously. 'That quiver . . . I felt it – the words – as I was reading it' (Deborah, on reading aloud 'Mysteriously Standing'); 'the words – certain words – jump out at you' (John, on 'The Pot Geranium'); 'Your read something and you can just turn – your body, your emotions – it takes your breath away you know' (Fay, on her response to Wharton's 'Mrs Manstey's View'); 'it seems to resonate, you feel it deep inside' (David, on 'The Liar'); 'It got into me' (Mary, on listening to Yeats's 'The Lake Isle of Innisfree'). Such responses are common to all the studies carried out in relation to Shared Reading: 'It has really hit me; right there [points to heart]'; 'The poem really zeroed in on my feelings, laid them bare'.[35] 'The poem just touched something in me.'[36] They attest to the frequency with which involuntary emotional, neo-physical connections happen at a level anterior to considered response. 'When a poem or story is read aloud, making every word and every line a close, vocal-emotional presence, the reader's response is likely to be situated in the body, as the biological substrate of an emotion, before it ever reaches mental awareness or consciously understood meaning.'[37] At the same time, as we saw in Part II, the voiced text, alive, near, intimate – the very thing which brings to life dormant inward matter – is also itself the secure centre. It 'grounds' or 'anchors' group members in the present, 'pulling'[38] them in to a space that is at once meditative (*It creates a stillness and peace in the room*), mindful (absorbed, attentive, immersed) and also feeling-ful, safely exposing readers to powerful memory. 'It wasn't in the past, it was going on at the time'; 'The poem kind of short-cut into a feeling when I was least expecting it. It just happened quite – suddenly'.[39] The literary material puts 'readers in touch and in place with resonant areas of deep human experience otherwise difficult to locate or recover, trigger[ing] access to subterranean or "underneath" experience in place of effort or guidance. Without the readers trying, [their] attention is "stabilised" and instantly redirected "from outside to inside", focussed on an inner dimension and interior sensation'.[40] Talk therapies, says van der Kolk, too often 'bypass the emotional-engagement system, encoded in visceral sensation, that is the foundation of who we are and instead focus narrowly on correcting "faulty thinking" and on suppressing unpleasant emotions and troublesome behaviours'.[41] Not *this* talk therapy, I am arguing. As my colleague in psychology, and collaborator on several Shared Reading studies, Rhiannon Corcoran puts it:

> Therapies such as CBT work through disciplined planned stages, outside of immediate experience, to prevent repetitive thought-patterns. The therapist says, 'Don't dwell on the bad stuff', 'Look forward – try not to look back'. Reading, by contrast, is an evolving process where breakthroughs into meaning happen from within an experience. The 'top-down' regulatory basis of CBT, where thinking is originally suggested by another and then taken on by the self, may be likely to produce only short-lived, 'un-owned' effects. Reading works from below upwards. The executive brain gets to work with genuine, spontaneous and 'owned' gut- or heart-responses and becomes involved in integrating them into models of the world.[42]

Reading starts where healing starts, in the body's gut- or heart-responses, touching off profound contact with hitherto denied or regretted or troubled experience, and giving it reality in the anchored here and now, prior to articulation.

But, as we saw in Part II, live reading does not merely 'hit' trouble: almost simultaneously, it holds, contains, 'thinks' it and thereby helps to release into conscious awareness aspects of being – painful emotion particularly – which might otherwise be passively suffered. The very distinction between bottom-up and top-down emotion and cognition begins to seem untenable. Or rather, to put it another way, literature and literary reading both model and foster the neural connectivity or 'cross-talk'[43] that characterizes an emotional life that is fully alive. Indeed, this is precisely how and why Shared Reading pivots between top-down talk and bottom-up 'visceral' approaches.

It does so in another way, too. 'The rational brain', to rehearse van der Kolk's central thesis, 'cannot *abolish* emotions, sensations or thoughts (such as living with a low-level sense of threat). . . . Understanding why you feel a certain way does not change *how* you feel'.[44] There is little to separate this bottom line from Freud's own. As Adam Phillips says, the very aim of the mother of all talk therapies, psychoanalysis, was to blow what van der Kolk calls the 'cover story', to allow people to hear their inner lives, what they really think and want, without feeling the need to 'pigeon-hole and padlock' them. 'There is nothing more defensive, Freud implies, than understanding what one is saying. The project of the unacceptable in oneself is to make itself known. Freud invented a therapeutic method [free association] in which this self could be overheard.'[45] EMDR is arguably itself an evolution of this invention, using the original trauma as the starting-point but essentially focused on 'stimulating and opening up the associative process'. But in addition to 'loosening up' shut-down psycho-biological matter, EDMR has the advantage, says van der Kolk, of allowing people to heal from trauma 'without verbal give-and-take with another person'.[46] This is especially valuable for people so traumatized as to be unable to engage in an open, trusting relationship with a therapist.

Analogously, in Shared Reading, as a psychiatrist running a reading group in a high secure hospital with widespread incidence of self-harm and chronic pain, once put it: 'The book [not the therapist] becomes the expert.'[47] Moreover, it does so without demanding the trust of the reader. 'You're not asked to respond personally', said one member of the chronic pain reading group, 'you just do'.[48]

Reading, neuroscience and emotion

Recent neuroscientific work in respect of literary reading is largely supportive of the central contention of this chapter: that literature has the power to galvanize stuckness. Vittorio Gallese, one of the scientists who discovered the mirror neuron phenomenon alluded to in Part II, proposes that reading fiction gives 'intimacy with a world we not only imagine, but literally embody'. As mirror neurons discharge both when a motor act is executed and when it is observed being performed by someone else, so, when perceiving others exhibiting emotion, the same brain areas are activated as when we subjectively experience the same emotion. Mirror neurons allow a direct form of 'action understanding' such that when we see someone expressing an emotional state, we can 'grasp its content without the need to reason explicitly about it'. This occurs through a mechanism of 'embodied simulation' or 'Feeling of Body' (FoB). Gallese offers FoB as an alternative to standard accounts of Theory of Mind or Mind-Reading.

> Embodied simulation is a mandatory, prerational, non-introspective process – that is, a physical, and not simply 'mental' experience of the mind, emotions, lived experiences and motor intentions of other people. [It] challenges the notion that interpersonal understanding consists solely of our explicitly attributing to others propositional attitudes like beliefs and desires, which we map as symbolic representations within our own minds. Embodied simulation creates internal non-linguistic 'representations' of the body-states associated with actions, emotions, and sensations [with the result that] we can map others' actions onto our own motor system, as well as others' emotions and sensations onto our own visceromotor and somatosensory systems.[49]

Gallese and Wojciehowski compare this model to Antonio Damasio's 'as-if body loop', which enables us to feel an emotional state 'as if the body were being activated and modified', rather than solely from 'actual' states,[50] though the relation of actual to imaginary is necessarily blurred by our bodily involvement in interpersonal relations. As the authors explain in a more recent essay: 'Our engagement with fictional characters is cognitively – and bodily – premediated by our life engagement, which provides the basic framing to navigate the world of fiction. . . . The same brain circuits that determine movement are "exploited" or "reused" to map the movements of others, both the real and the fictional ones.' In turn (corroborating the evidence and endorsing the propositions of Part II of this book), narrated material can at once 'awake bodily memories in the reader's mind' and 'premediate life experience, as our engagement with fictional characters provides clues and perspectives that can affect how we cope with life's challenges'. 'The border separating real and imaginary worlds appears much less sharp and clear when viewed from a neuroscientific perspective.'[51]

The concept of embodied cognition, which has gained strong currency in literary studies in recent years, shares affinity with David Miall's prescient insistence (three decades earlier) on the centrality of emotion in literary response, shifting the emphasis from the cognitive to the affective in accounting for literature's power to reshape inner schemata.[52] Gallese's emphasis on the bodily nature of intersubjectivity in his account of literary response, influenced as it is by the work of Stern,[53] adds a neuro dimension to the pre- or non-verbal vitality affects engendered by shared literary reading, which were the concluding concern of Part II. But the brain-body model of literary affect has also been substantiated by recent work on the psychophysiology of responses to poetry (rather than fiction alone). Adapting approaches to music reception, this work shows poetry's power to induce 'peak emotional experiences, including subjectively reported chills and objectively reported goosebumps'. Poetry from the eighteenth to the twentieth century, some self-selected, some selected by the experimenters and listened to via professional (commercial) audio-recordings, was shown to trigger 'not only mild affective responses but also the most intense ones'. This 'very strong effect on the bodies and brains of listeners' was not only found to be consistent with the much more extensively studied affective power of listening to music. An unexpected finding (given the assumption that poetry the listeners knew and chose themselves would evoke the most intense responses) was that chills and goosebumps were elicited as much by the unfamiliar as the familiar stimuli.[54] This relates directly to Corcoran's recognition of the power of live reading to trigger 'active happenings and unpredictable events' in place of 'undemanding and convenient defaults'. 'Routine must be deviated from and uncertainty tolerated, [removing] the facility to rely on a safe system. We cannot predict and so cannot control our responses. Our own experiences are re-felt or reviewed in a way which challenges habitual emotions or recovers them in a new form.'[55] Moreover, the 'chills and goosebumps' study found that intense arousal coincided in 'a remarkably consistent pattern' with instances where the poetry's formal composition – rhyme, rhythm and structural organization – were foregrounded.[56] This invokes the body of work on 'communicative musicality' as a biological substrate of literary response, which we encountered in the last chapter, as well as endorsing Miall's and Kuiken's rationale in relation to the key role of defamiliarization in literary response. It also firmly intersects with other cognitive neuroscientific studies which are beginning to comprehend the complex neural connectivities involved in literary reading. Jacobs's (albeit speculative) model for the neurocognitive poetics of literary response, based on existing state-of-the-art evidence, posits that familiar elements of literary texts (words, images, situations, sociocultural codes whose meanings are transparent) are implicitly processed predominantly by the left hemisphere reading network. These are the brain regions which have been identified as consistently and automatically engaged during reading to enable effortless fluency (measured by a high rate of words per minute and undisturbed eye movement control), and, which, it is supposed, provide the conditions for more complex and effortful processes of inference and interpretation carried out by right hemisphere networks. By contrast, when non-standard elements or semantic ambiguities are encountered, slower reading rates and decelerated or irregular (fixated, regressive) eye movement patterns indicate activation of the right hemisphere's associative (non-literal, intuitive, connection-forming, creative) networks. 'The reader is now in a "poetic mode" of tacit evaluative processing . . . not only (automatically) recognizing words but "seeing", "hearing", "smelling" them.'[57] This model is supported by studies of the effect on brain activation of classic Shakespearean foregrounding (specifically the conversion of one part of speech – adjective, noun, verb – to another, for metaphorical compression, as in 'A father and a gracious aged man: him have you *madded*'[58]). A shift in activation was likewise found from left homophone structures activated by typical language tasks, to right hemisphere additional (non-verbal, visual and emotion) networks, 'as if Shakespeare's language, thus engaging multiple levels of brain activity, were creating a three-dimensional space behind the eyes'.[59] There was evidence, too, that Shakespeare's violation of grammatical and semantic norms excited brain activity which at once accepted the sense of the metaphor, while also registering its strangeness, thereby simultaneously blocking default responses and raising attention and alertness to novel connections and meanings.[60]

These preliminary findings of the power of literary language to baulk simple automaticity and galvanize new neural pathways and emotion networks are particularly relevant to chronic pain in which, as we have seen, the nervous system produces persistent 'pain pathways'. Continuous or repetitive stimulation of pain receptors leads to changes in neuronal structure which result in hyperexcitable pain sensitization. This hardwiring of neural pathways is influenced by psychological stressors such as anxiety and depression, which accentuate pain intensity and affect a person's capacity to tolerate pain. Such stressors, as noted in Part I, are a particular risk factor in the transition from acute to chronic pain. Thus, intervening at an optimum stage in the neuroplasticity of the pain brain might be crucial. 'Theoretically, if the pathophysiological changes during this transition could be prevented or reversed, we would be able to prevent or minimise the development of chronic pain in practice.'[61] Significantly, in this regard, one recent neuroscientific study of literary reading has found that 'processing poetic content requires a switch away from stored representations' by modulating brain regions 'associated with the ability to represent and manipulate fluid, flexible meanings'. The authors propose that literary reading may entrain, therefore, a more dynamic, responsive and less rigid thinking style. As maladaptive beliefs and dysfunctional connectivity (linked to depression as well as chronic pain) together help sustain mental health difficulties, it is possible that reading poetry and fiction may 'divert individuals away from processing their struggles via ingrained and ineffective channels [and help] scaffold functional beliefs that cannot so easily sustain worries, troubles and negative automatic thoughts'.[62]

*

Finally, as a mini thought experiment, I wish, at the near-close of this book, to consider the relevance to this book's concerns of recent neuroscience which, though unrelated to literature or reading, potentially offers an existing rationale for the contention that Shared Reading has the potential to release emotional stuckness.

In *How Emotions Are Made,* Lisa Feldman Barrett advances a theory of emotion within the scientific tradition of 'construction', 'which holds that your experiences and behaviours are created in the moment by biological processes within your brain and body'. Barrett opposes this theory to what she calls 'the classical view of emotion'. According to the latter, emotions are evolutionary legacies, once vital for survival, which are now 'a fixed component of our biological nature', each with its own 'defining underlying pattern in the brain and body'. (Sadness activates a particular set of neurons – the 'sadness circuit'; so it is with anger, surprise and so on). Scientific investigation, however (and Barrett bases her thesis on systematic meta-analysis of published studies over the last twenty years as well as research over the past century), suggests otherwise. These experiments 'revealed no consistent, specific [physiological] fingerprints . . . for different emotions. [Rather] on different occasions, in different contexts, in different studies, within the same individuals and across different individuals, *the same emotion category involves different bodily responses.* Variation not uniformity is the norm'. This does not mean, says Barrett, that 'emotions are an illusion or that bodily responses are random'. It *does* mean, firstly, that 'emotion is not a *thing* but a category, and an emotion category has tremendous variety', and, secondly, that 'emotions are in fact made and not triggered'. 'Emotions are not built-in but made from more basic parts. . . . They emerge as a combination of the physical properties of your body [and] a flexible brain that wires itself to whatever environment it develops in.' Thus, in opposition to the conventional stimulus-response model, Barrett proposes that emotion is 'made' according to the same neuroanatomical principles upon which all other perceptions are constructed. When faced with new sensory input, brain neurons sift through past experiences seeking those most similar to the current one. 'Which combination of my past experiences provides the closest match to this particular situation?' The brain generates multiple 'best guesses' from its vast network of neural connections of what is happening and of what to do next. 'In every waking moment', faced with the random incoming data of the world ('the light, vibrations and chemicals that become sights, sounds and smells'), the brain 'uses your past experience to construct a hypothesis – a simulation – to guide your actions'. Simulation happens 'so invisibly and automatically' that the activity of the senses (vision, hearing) 'seem like reflexes rather than constructions', where 'scientific evidence shows that what we see, hear, touch, taste, smell are largely simulations of the world, not reactions to it'. Barrett goes on:

> Your brain uses the same process to make meaning of the sensations from *inside your body* . . . the commotion arising from your heartbeat, breathing and other internal movements. . . . From your brain's perspective, your body is just another source of sensory input . . . purely physical sensations inside your body have no objective psychological meaning. . . . An emotion is your brain's *creation* of what your bodily sensations mean. Emotions are not reactions to the world. You are not a passive receiver of sensory input but an active constructor of your emotions.

Thus, just as 'through simulation, prediction, hypothesis, your brain constructs the world it experiences', so too it constructs its emotional reality. These constructions are not merely arbitrary in a brain that is modelling a reality whose sensory input it is steeped in and awash with. As the brain models the world, the world wires the brain, such that 'the dividing line between brain and world is permeable, perhaps non-existent'. The notion of neural footprints has no place, asserts Barrett, in a process so dynamic. 'The human brain . . . is organised for variation. . . . Ever-changing populations of neurons form and dissolve in milliseconds, so that single neurons participate in different situations, modelling a variable and only partly predictable world.'

At the same time, the brain can only work with the simulations it can generate. If your repertoire is rich and wide, 'your brain [has] many more options for predicting, categorising and perceiving emotion' and for constructing 'fine-grained' instances of emotion 'that are finely tailored to fit each specific situation'. Central to Barrett's thesis is the possibility that a constructionist model of emotion can foster a view of human beings as 'architects' of their own experience rather than merely 'reactive animals', and that this might have particular application for understanding illnesses (including chronic pain and depression) in which emotion is strongly implicated. 'People who exhibit higher emotional granularity go to the doctor less frequently, use medication less frequently and spend fewer days hospitalised with illness.' 'The key is to gain new emotion concepts and hone existing ones. . . . New experiences [Barrett includes book-reading] provoke the brain to combine concepts to form new ones, changing your conceptual system proactively' and creating awareness of 'which ones to use when'.[63]

There is a self-evident connection here with the theories from reading psychology we encountered in Part II which posit literary texts as offering just the kind of enriched and extended models and schema for experience which Barrett proposes as necessary tools for a meaningful and healthy life. Indeed, it is in part on the basis that 'simulation is the default mode for all mental activity',[64] as Barrett puts it, that Oatley bases his argument for 'fiction as simulation' in which personal truths and emotions can be explored and understood. 'The essence of [simulation] is that mental life is constructive. The machinery of cognitive construction, the reader's share, is within everyone.'[65]

Moreover, Barrett's 'recipe' for 'the easiest way' to enlarge emotional understanding – 'learn new words [since] words seed your concepts, concepts drive your predictions'[66] – has a strong synergy both with the importance, as we saw in Part I, of addressing the issue of alexithymia in people experiencing chronic pain and associated health problems, and with the expansion of vocabulary and a language for emotional experience which we saw Shared Reading providing in Part II.

But the implications of this theory for the process of Shared Reading seem to me to be more profound, and encouraging, still. The fact that 'emotions are not reactions' but a meaning which the brain constructs out of the dynamic between sensory input in the here and now and past experiences means that they are also not fixed or inexorable. 'Heart rate changes are inevitable, their emotional meaning is not.' The exciting idea from a therapeutic perspective, and especially in relation to the stimulus of literature in Shared Reading, is the potential for '[different] kinds of meaning from the same sensory input'.[67] So, for example, when a poem takes a person 'right back into' an experience or memory or thought, as we saw repeatedly in Part II, there is a possibility that the meaning of that experience, through the medium of the poem and its language, can be fundamentally changed – neurally, biologically reshaped. One is not stuck with one way of seeing that experience, or oneself, or the world as a result of it, but is open to a rewired vision or perspective, catalysed by the poem's own. Moreover, if emotions are created in the instant by biological processes within one's brain and body, then even the passing emotions that take place in a reading group have a chance of dislodging stuck mentalities by assigning new meanings to old experiences, most especially insofar as they stimulate 'emotional granularity' – the capacity to conceive and categorize emotion with precision using a finely grained vocabulary – which further enhances neural mobility.[68]

This possibility of here-and-now change connects with two key ideas with which the individual reading case studies concluded in Chapter 8. Firstly, the notion of the creative present, as, not 'merely a fleeting and passing moment of now, which is constantly running out or lacking any duration' but as 'an affirmative and creative texture which enables and facilitates change'. Such a possibility is of particular emancipatory value to people living in the relative stagnation and recurring succession of chronic time which we encountered in Part II. Barrett's thesis points to the same conclusion as therapy for chronic illness in practice: 'As even the most repetitive action or experience entails asymmetries, is never the same in any of its repeats', instead of chronicity amounting to assumed sterile 'unproductive seriality', repetition and recurrence can acquire a 'transformative' potential.[69] Secondly, there is an analogy with the psychoanalytic situation as Levine (after Bion) conceives it. 'A "memory" [created out of] a here-and-now present day interaction in the analysis, may work to dynamically "patch over" a "hole" or "psychic void" left in the wake of previous pre-verbal or psychic trauma.' While the newly created memory of meaning 'cannot change the reality' of the traumatic happening or influence, it can 'help initiate or reinforce psychic structures'[70] (as well as, Barrett suggests, neural ones) which are essential to emotional and mental health.

Such 'remediation'[71] is provided by the psychoanalyst, as we saw in Chapter 8, within the context of the psychoanalytical relationship which self-consciously offers itself as filling the 'hole' created by failed environmental provision in the past. Likewise, in Shared Reading, the 'here and now' relationship with the literary text, which has power to create new emotional meanings, is nurtured, as Chapter 9 demonstrated, in the context of a personalizing community in which 'inner lives come out together'.[72] This, as much as the literary text itself, might be critical therapeutically. 'When we look beyond the specific symptoms', says van der Kolk, almost all emotional suffering that results in illness involves 'trouble in creating workable or satisfying relationships' and thus a breakdown in our species' 'most powerful survival strategy', social collaboration. 'Our relationship maps are implicit', early 'etched' into the areas of the brain devoted to emotion and memory. They 'are not reversible simply by understanding how they are created'. They require later experiences which 'explore other ways to connect in relationships' and which make it possible to '(re)learn intimacy and mutual trust with fellow human beings'. 'If you carry a memory of having felt safe with somebody long ago, the traces of that earlier affection can be reactivated in attuned relationships when you are an adult.'[73] In illustrating how her theory of constructed emotion dismantles the separation between the environment 'out there' and the 'in here' of the brain, Barrett cites her experience of working as a therapist with college-aged women who were abused in childhood, and whose emotional suffering could only be resolved when their brains ceased 'to model a hostile world'.[74]

It is both instructive and alarming to note, in this context, that in Jaak Panksepp's chapter on 'Love and the Social Bond' in *Affective Neuroscience*, he explains that 'the first neurochemical system that was found to exert a powerful inhibitory effect on separation distress was the brain opioid system'. He goes on: 'It is now clear that positive social interactions derive part of their pleasure from the release of opioids in the brain' and that there are 'strong similarities between the dynamics of opiate addiction and social dependence':

> It is tempting to hypothesize that one reason certain people become addicted to external opiates [such as morphine and heroin] is because they are able to [experience] gratification similar to that normally achieved by the socially induced release of endogenous [internal] opioids . . . to pharmacologically induce the positive feeling of connectedness that others derive from social interactions. Is it any wonder that these people even become intensely attached (classically conditioned) to the paraphernalia associated with their drug experiences, or that addicts tend to become socially isolated, except when they are approaching withdrawal and seeking more drugs?

It is almost breathtaking to think that, at the time Panksepp was writing (in 1998) of the 'enormous psychiatric importance' of early social bonding and how 'if inadequately established, the organism can suffer severe consequences for the rest of its life',[75] people already vulnerable to chronic pain through insecure attachments (as we saw in Chapter 4) were being criminally encouraged in a drug addiction to which those very attachment issues also left them deeply vulnerable. The thinking cited in this chapter collectively and strenuously endorses interventions in chronic pain and its associated symptoms which rest on what Barrett's neuroscience of emotion advocates: 'a radically different view of what it means to be a human being'.[76]

Afterword

I close this book by urging literary reading for people suffering from chronic pain for two principal reasons.

The first reason is almost wholly a practical one. In a situation where the burden of chronic pain and associated mental health problems is huge and growing, and where research points to the need for a range of psychosocial treatments which readily combine with one another in a multi-intervention integrated pain management programme, Shared Reading offers one such highly flexible intervention. The model is easily and inexpensively replicable. It is currently delivered through an international model which can be multiplied at will for the modest cost of training Reader Leaders. This training can be, and in many clinical contexts currently is, accessed by health professionals – mental health providers, clinical psychologists, physiotherapists, nurses, GPs, and so on. It can be tailored to different resources, needs, contexts; it can last a few weeks or a few months; it can be offered weekly or every day, and be delivered in person and online. Shared Reading also pairs well with therapies currently established as chronic pain treatments both because, as we have seen, it is affined in orientation to these interventions and, arguably, brings together the best of traditional talk therapies with the best of meditation-based or body-oriented practices. In a recent innovation, a mindfulness therapist has tried to reciprocally maximize the effects of meditation and Shared Reading by incorporating both into a contemporary therapeutic programme for war veterans with a diagnosis of PTSD with attendant chronic pain symptoms. The rationale for this exploratory programme is that *the tendency towards experiential avoidance (in which subjects believe they are unable to maintain contact with unwanted internal experiences and create habitual responses in hopes of escaping or changing such experiences) has potential to be reduced through the 'titration' (measured quantity or dosage) of emotional contact that Shared Reading facilitates*. Early evidence is suggesting that affective experience is shifting in the expected direction as a result of this programme. Similar reasoning underlies the successful long-term delivery of a Shared Reading programme for patients in a secure psychiatric hospital, where self-harm and chronic pain combine in a complex symptomology, as a *primer* for formal therapy.

> *They lack connection with their own emotions. A patient might describe a feeling but not actually put themselves in it emotionally, because that would be too difficult to tolerate. Not connecting – it's protective. So when a patient says the reading group has made them 'care about things' that's real progress. Both self-harm and chronic pain are related to patients finding it hard to articulate their feelings or actually know what their feelings are. This lack of emotional vocabulary is very serious because one aspect of their self-injury and pain is chronic feelings of emptiness. A lot of patients' behaviours and symptoms are about wanting to fill this emptiness and to check they are still here. I thought that if my patients attended the reading group, they could start to think, instead of reacting, 'What's this hole inside me?', 'Can I fill that hole in a different way?'*

I urge the adoption of Shared Reading in full awareness of the problematic social prescribing context, detailed at the close of Chapter 1, in which such provision would be likely to operate most of the time. As we saw there, community-level non-clinical activities can potentially play a critical role in de-medicalizing care and reaching marginalized groups. The consensus is that a sustainable model will require strong collaboration between health and social care providers, local authorities, cultural, educational and leisure organizations and an integrated and cooperative approach.[1] But the examples I cite above suggest that something more than a robust infrastructure alone, crucial though that is, might be needful. In these instances, a mindfulness practitioner and psychiatrist have integrated Shared Reading into their own practice of healthcare. This is not mere 'sign-posting' *in place of* a biopsychosocial model of care but closer to a revitalizing of the latter. Insofar as literary reading engenders a more personal interaction and orientation within a formal caregiving context, it can be regarded in these instances as a kind of equivalent of the training in 'micro-practices' which Felicity Thomas developed for GPs to build trust and create 'space for the patients to be listened to and heard'.[2] In many ways, the model of Shared Reading provision that has absorbed this book exhibits both forms of integration outlined above: on the one hand, Shared Reading is a strategic part of the 'treatment package' provided by the pain clinic; on the other, the consultants carefully assess the appropriateness of referring patients based on their individual needs, suggesting 'taster' attendances rather than long-term commitment in the first instance. Importantly, too, the health providers in this case were also closely involved in the research that went into understanding why and how literary reading was 'working' for their patients. This not only helped them, as we witnessed intermittently in Part II, to see their patients in a new or different way; it led to reflections on their own practice as well as on the value of literature in relation to their own lives. For example:

We've got our perceived self, our hoped-for self, and it seems intuitively true to say that the further apart your hoped-for self and your perceived self are then the more trouble you're in. Could it be that by exploring characters and emotions in books, you're able to . . . perhaps bring them closer together, your hoped-for self and your perceived self. It's a reformulation.

Something more than the value of a literary health intervention seems to be at stake here, however, something which bears more generally on the place or role of literature when it collaborates in thinking or practice around health and medicine. Let me hold open this idea alongside two recent accounts of the positioning of literature in relation to two disciplines of key relevance to the project of this book: Medical Humanities and Psychoanalysis.

In 'Literature in the Critical Medical Humanities', Angela Woods and James Rákóczi ask, 'What is happening to literature, literariness, the literary text and the literary scholar as they get caught up in collaborative, interdisciplinary, critical and health-related projects?' From the interviews the authors conducted with scholars thus 'caught up', they found that '"the literary" was most often invoked . . . as an orientation, approach or sensibility'. (For the sake of compactness, I draw together quotations and comments relating to several interviewees.)

> What literary studies gives to critical medical humanities is a fine ear for messiness and contradictions and narratives that don't make sense and a capacity to 'attune' to illness and life's possibilities more thoroughly and attentively. The value of literature lies in its capacity to contain mess without resolution, holding on to inconsistences and contradiction, allowing proooooooo to unfold rather than be prodotorminod, and lotting oonoopto be emergent rather than rigidly set - qualities recognised as particularly valuable in contexts where the complexities of illness experience and of interdisciplinary collaboration were in play.

While these recognitions gave literary scholars a 'renewed faith in the literary text', at the same time it was acknowledged that

> Doing English within an interdisciplinary medical humanities project is . . . a very different kind of endeavour which somewhat counter-intuitively *decentres* the text and forms of distinctly *literary* criticism.[3]

Now here is Vera Camden, in her introduction to the *Cambridge Companion to Literature and Psychoanalysis*:

> If psychoanalysis is a practice that offers amelioration of human suffering, literature is the source of that practice. [It is] a companionate

marriage . . . between two mentalities, two languages of human meaning. . . . The significance of this bond has often been elided in academic as well as clinical discussions of psychoanalytic theory. Pierre Bayard puts it this way: 'As it is often practised, the psychoanalytical approach to texts places knowledge on the side of psychoanalysis and not on that of literature. In doing so, it risks diminishing literature and underestimating literature's own ability to produce knowledge.' Against this trend, [this volume] places literature at the centre of psychoanalytic thought avowing that psychoanalysis itself derives life and purpose from literature. . . . [It] places literature before psychoanalysis, foregrounding the work of poets, novelists, playwrights, film-makers, comics artists, and other creators as foundational to psychoanalysis then and now.[4]

Woods's and Rákóczi's study resoundingly echoes the ways in which we have seen literature matter to the readers encountered in this book – by offering, that is, a richly porous container or means of 'holding' unresolved and often intractable life matter, including, though by no means confined to, the experience of illness. Camden's project gives retrospective affirmation to this book's reliance on the interdependence of literature and psychoanalysis to help account for the therapeutic power of fiction and poetry, as illustrated by the case studies in Part II. What strikes me about both of these accounts, however, is the sense of the relative *precarity* of the status of the literary text, even when it is protected by literary specialists, and even as it is the acknowledged source of what is prized: knowledge, or sensibility, or a fine ear. 'The medical humanities offers "a huge opportunity to show why literary studies matter" but literary studies "can only really be effective . . . if it understands its own value".'[5] The positioning of literature as vulnerable to being diminished, decentred, underestimated, even because of the very subtlety and implicitness of its influence, casts into a newly bold and radical light The Reader's project, from the very outset, of placing the literary text at the very *centre* – first and before all – at every weekly session. One unexpected consequence of simply, yet riskily, doing so – beyond the relative protection of academe, exporting this crucial 'language of human meaning' into the wider world – is that the renewed 'faith' in literary studies, which Woods and Rákóczi discovered and which Camden champions, might be further reinvigorated outside-in, through bearing witness to the value of literature for people, and those who care for them, who are struggling in ordinary life.

This brings me to the second (ontological) reason for recommending Shared Reading: the need for meaning – meaning that is new, revised or rediscovered. This need has crossed this book at every turn, precisely because the absence of meaning, however it has come to be lost, has the power to contribute to the development of chronic pain and is certainly likely to prolong it. 'Pain, why they have pain. It's usually very similar', says a resident of the pain centre in Jean Jackson's study: 'they lost control someplace'.[6] Nothing, says Gendlin, is as debilitating as losing direct touch with the inner life, 'with our own personally important experiencing' such that the latter's intrinsic meaning is unavailable. Yet, Gendlin suggests, this is more the rule than not in modern Western culture.

> The chief malaise of our society is that it allows so little pause and gives so little specifying response and interpersonal communion to our experiencing, so that we must much of the time pretend that we are only what we seem externally, and that our meanings are only the objective references and the logical meanings of our words.[7]

Shared Reading, as we saw in Chapter 9, offers just such an interpersonal space and protected pause for pondering authentic internal meanings. But, crucially, it also offers that space over time. This is important not only in view of recent evidence that long-term therapeutic interventions are more effective for chronic (depressive) conditions than short-term ones.[8] Such outcomes perhaps themselves derive from the freedom to grow in accord with a personal 'rhythm' or 'pulse' of change – not 'progressing on time' but 'being *in* time', and '*in* progress, unfinished'. Literary reading, as we saw in Part II, can be especially valuable in activating 'an individualised temporality of change' which at once resists the damaging influence of chronicity, conceptually and experientially ('As every category affects the thing it is used to categorise . . . a temporal perception of "chronicity" entails creating "chronic" kinds of patients'[9]), and allows for the kind of complex transformation, both in the moment and across time, which is discontinuous, provisional, neither preconceived nor straightforwardly linear. This is why it is important that the stimulus – the book, story or poem – is still available to the reader even when the group is not. Just as Gendlin's 'focusing' method (mentioned in Chapter 5) is designed as a form of self-help for those who do not have access to other forms of aid – counsellors, therapy, pastors, doctors, friends, family – so the ancient technology of literature can be considered a protean form of life support.

More importantly, this support is neutral, non-partisan and without expectation. The analogy I have in mind here is Jean Jackson's account of the value of her own discipline in respecting the integrity of chronic pain as it is individually experienced. Writing of the pitfalls of narrating another's pain, she specifies the advantage of anthropology's orientation over that of biomedicine and social science, where narratives of pain are inevitably influenced by the positivist goals of medico-scientific professionals seeking to understand, diagnose and alleviate pain. 'This is not the goal of ethnography', Jackson says.

> The ultimate goal in narrating another person's pain is an optimal understanding that leads to optimal narration. . . . Therapeutic suggestions that are at odds with the sufferer's beliefs [should not] distract from the main purpose, which is to temporarily shelve such judgments and represent another person's experience accurately and comprehensively, to represent another person's reality, from whatever moral world that person inhabits.[10]

Viewed from this perspective, literary language is arguably the ideal 'narrator' of painful experience. Not only is the reader free to choose the work which best tells their own story – or more usually, free to allow the work (non-coercively) to choose *them*. The book or poem also has no agenda in relation to the reader, nor any knowledge of or interest in their pain. On the contrary, imaginative works, said Kenneth Burke, are improvised 'answers to questions posed by the situation in which they arose'. Humans, with 'the same neural, muscular and biological structure . . . have left their records from past ages' of 'the various strategies for sizing up situations'. It is because literary writing stays so urgently and exclusively close to the messy relations of particularized individual life ('whatever moral world that person inhabits'), that it has, paradoxically, what Burke calls 'public'[11] value. At once uniquely disinterested and uniquely engaged, literature is that rare thing in our culture: a specialist discourse that is open to everyone, and always there, anywhere, anytime, whenever you need it.

Notes

Chapter 1

1 P. R. Keefe, *Empire of Pain* (London: Picador, 2021), 4–5.

2 Centre for Disease Control and Prevention, 17 November 2021, https://www.cdc.gov/nchs/nvss/vsrr/drug-overdose-data.htm (accessed 16 September 2023).

3 K. Humphreys, et al., 'Responding to the Opioid Crisis in North America and Beyond: Recommendations of the Stanford-*Lancet* Commission', *Lancet* 399, no. 10324 (2022): 555–604.

4 A. Kleinman, *The Illness Narratives* (New York: Basic Books, 1988), 73.

5 G. E. Engel, 'Need for a New Medical Model', *Science* 196, no. 4286 (1977): 129–36.

6 G. E. Engel, 'Clinical Application of the Biopsychosocial Model', *American Journal of Psychiatry* 135, no. 5 (1980): 535–44, 535, 537.

7 R. Melzack, 'From the Gate to the Neuromatrix', *Pain* 82 (1999): S121–S126.

8 S. M. Meints and R. R. Edwards, 'Psychosocial Contributions to Chronic Pain Outcomes', *Progress Neuropsychopharmacology and Biological Psychiatry* 20, no. 87 (2018): 168–82, 168. For wide-ranging interdisciplinary perspectives on the multi-dimensional characteristics of pain, see S. P. van Rysewyk, ed., *Meanings of Pain*, 3 vols. (Cham: Springer, 2019–2022).

9 S. N. Raja, et al., 'Revised International Association for Study of Pain Definition of Pain', *Pain* 161, no. 9 (2020): 1976–82, 1976.

10 When quoting, as I do here, directly from primary data gathered for the study, I use italics to distinguish testimony from participants and collaborators in the study from quotations from published sources.

11 M. C. Lee and I. Tracey, 'Imaging Pain', *British Journal of Anaesthesia* 111, no. 13 (2013): 64–72, 64.

12 S. E. E. Mills, et al., 'Chronic Pain: Review of its Epidemiology', *British Journal of Anaesthesia* 123, no. 2 (2019): E273–E283.

13 Lee and Tracey, 'Imaging Pain', 64.

14 NHS Digital Prescriptions dispensed in the community, statistics for England, 2006–2016, 29 June 2017, http://digital.nhs.uk/catalogue/PUB30014 (accessed 25 June 2024).

15 C. Dowrick and A. Frances, 'Medicalising Unhappiness', *British Medical Journal* 347 (2013): f7140. Christopher Dowrick was a key collaborator on the reading and depression study cited below, n. 16. I discuss the implications of the paper cited here more fully in J. Billington, *Is Literature Healthy?* (Oxford: Oxford University Press, 2016), 1–3.

16 J. Billington et al., *An Investigation into the Therapeutic Benefits of Reading in Relation to Depression and Well-being* (Liverpool: Liverpool Health Inequalities Research Institute, 2010). For further published material arising from this study, see Chapter 5, n. 3.

17 See n. 14.

18 B. Barr et al., 'Trends in Mental Health Inequalities in England During a Period of Recession, Austerity and Welfare Reform 2004 to 2013', *Social Science and Medicine* 147 (2015): 324–31.

19 D. Tsimpida et al., 'Unravelling the Dynamics of Mental Health Inequalities in England', *SSM—Population Health* 26 (2024): 101669.

20 F. Thomas et al., 'Moral Narratives and Mental Health', *Palgrave Communications* 4 (2018): 39.

21 A key aim, in fact, of the NHS's Implementing the 5 Year Forward View for Mental Health, 2017, https://www.england.nhs.uk/publication/implementing-the-fyfv-for-mental-health/ (accessed 25 June 2024).

22 Thomas et al., 'Moral Narratives and Mental Health'.

23 S. von Peter, 'The Temporality of "Chronic" Mental Illness', *Culture, Medicine and Psychiatry* 34 (2010): 13–28, 13–15.

24 L. Manderson and C. Smith-Morris, 'Introduction: Chronicity and the Experience of Illness', in , *Chronic Conditions, Fluid States: Chronicity and the Anthropology of Illness,* ed. Manderson and Smith-Morris (New Brunswick: Rutgers University Press, 2010), 1–18, 4–5.

25 A. K. Schaffner, *Exhaustion: A History* (New York: Columbia University Press, 2016), 8, 128.

26 Manderson and Smith-Morris, *Chronic Conditions, Fluid States: Chronicity and the Anthropology of Illness*, 10.

27 A. Ehrenberg, *The Weariness of Self: Diagnosing the History of Depression in the Contemporary Age* (Montreal and Kingston: McGill-Queen's University Press, 2009), 9, 185.

28 B. C. Han, *The Palliative Society*, trans. D. Steuer (Cambridge: Polity, 2021), 11.

29 Manderson and Smith, *Chronic Conditions, Fluid States: Chronicity and the Anthropology of Illness*, 6.

30 Manderson and Smith, *Chronic Conditions, Fluid States: Chronicity and the Anthropology of Illness*, 10.

31 R. White et al., 'Counterflows for Mental Well-being: What High-Income Countries Can Learn from Low and Middle-income Countries', *International Review of Psychiatry* 26, no. 5 (2014): 602–6.

32 R. R. Edwards, et al., 'Role of Psychosocial Processes in Development and Maintenance of Chronic Pain', *Journal of Pain* 17, no. 9 (2016): T70–T92, T72.

33 S. M. Banks and R. D. Kerns, 'Explaining High Rates of Depression in Chronic Pain', *Psychological Bulletin* 119, no. 1 (1996): 95–110.

34 M. J. Bair, et al., 'Depression and Pain Comorbidity', *Archives of Internal Medicine* 163, no. 20 (2003): 2433–45.

35 Thomas et al., 'Moral Narratives and Mental Health'.

36 D. Koesling and C. Bozzaro, 'Chronic Pain as a Blind Spot in the Diagnosis of a Depressed Society', *Medicine, Health Care and Philosophy* 25, no. 4 (2022): 671–80, 671, 676–8.

37 *Diagnostic and Statistical Manual of Mental Disorders* (DSM-5) (Washington, DC: American Psychiatric Association, 2013).

38 M. Haack, et al., 'Sleep Deficiency and Chronic Pain', *Neuropsychopharmacology* 45, no. 1 (2020): 205–16.

39 T. Mallick-Searle, et al., 'Pain and Function in Chronic Musculoskeletal Pain', *Journal of Multidisciplinary Healthcare* 14 (2021): 335–44.

40 C. A. Lee, et al., 'Change of Weight and Chronic Low Back Pain', *International Journal of Environmental Research and Public Health* 18, no. 8 (2021): 3969.

41 M. A. Hadi, et al., 'Impact of Chronic Pain on Quality of Life', *Journal of Patient Experience* 6, no. 2 (2019): 133–41.

42 S. T. Fiske and S. E. Taylor, *Social Cognition*, 2nd edn (New York : McGraw-Hill, 1991), 23.

43 S. F. Maier and M. E. P. Seligman, 'Learned Helplessness', *Journal of Experimental Psychology: General* 105, no. 1 (1976): 3–46, 13, 6.

44 T. Rudy, et al., 'Chronic Pain and Depression', *Pain* 35 (1988): 129–40, 101.

45 M. G. Pereira, et al., 'Quality of Life in Chronic Pain', *PsyCh Journal* 10, no. 2 (2021): 283–94.

46 A. T. Beck, 'Cognitive Model of Depression and Its Neurobiological Correlates', *American Journal of Psychiatry* 105, no. 8 (2008): 969–77, 970.

47 Beck, 'Cognitive Model of Depression', 970.

48 Banks and Kerns, 'Explaining High Rates of Depression in Chronic Pain', 105.

49 Beck, 'Cognitive Model of Depression', 971.

50 A. T. Beck, *Depression: Causes and Treatment* (Philadelphia: University of Pennsylvania Press, 1967).

51 As we shall see shortly, the pre-frontal cortex (PFC), central to the perception of and emotional response to pain, undergoes distinct grey matter changes in both volume and connectivity, which can hardwire neuronal pathways between brain areas associated with negative thoughts and emotions and pain perception. (See p. 19.)

52 M. Von Korff, et al., 'First Onset of Common Pain Symptoms', *Pain* 55, no. 2 (1993): 251–8; M. J. G. Marloes, et al., 'Longitudinal Association Between Pain, Depression and Anxiety', *Journal of Psychosomatic Research* 78, no. 1 (2015): 64–70; G. J. G. Asmundson and J. Katz, 'Co-Occurrence of Anxiety Disorders and Chronic Pain', *Depression and Anxiety* 26, no. 10 (2009): 888–901.

53 Mills, et al., 'Chronic Pain: A Review'.

54 K. Kroenke, et al., 'Antidepressant Therapy and Pain Self-management in Patients with Depression and Musculoskeletal Pain', *Journal of American Medical Association* 301, no. 20 (2009): 2099–110; S. Rej, et al., 'Treating Concurrent Chronic Low Back Pain and Depression', *Pain Medicine* 15, no. 7 (2014): 1154–62.

55 R. R. Edwards, et al., 'Pain, Catastrophizing, and Depression', *Nature Reviews Rheumatology* 7, no. 4 (2011): 216–24; A. D. Wasan, et al., 'Association Between Negative Affect and Opioid Analgesia in Patients with Discogenic Low Back Pain', *Pain* 117, no. 3 (2005): 450–61.

56 A. Wasan, et al., 'Diminished Opioid Analgesia, Increased Opioid Misuse in Patients with Chronic Low Back Pain', *Anesthesiology* 123, no. 4 (2015): 861–72.

57 D. C. Turk, et al., 'Outcome Domains for Chronic Pain', *Pain* 137, no. 2 (2008): 276–85.

58 Mills, et al., 'Chronic Pain: A Review'.

59 M. J. L. Sullivan, et al., 'Catastrophizing and Pain', *Clinical Journal of Pain* 17, no. 1 (2001): 52–64; F. J. Keefe, et al., 'Relationship of Gender to Pain: Role of Catastrophizing', *Pain* 87, no. 3 (2000): 325–34; R. R. Edwards, et al., 'Catastrophizing and Pain', *Arthritis and Rheumatism* 55, no. 2 (2006): 325–32.

60 M. K. Nicholas, et al., 'Depressive Symptoms in Patients with Chronic Pain', *Medical Journal of Australia* 190, no. 7 (2009): S66–70.

61 R. Severeijns, et al., 'Pain Catastrophizing and General Health Status', *Pain* 99, no. 1 (2002): 367–76.

62 R. R. Edwards, et al., 'Psychosocial Processes in Chronic Pain', T79.

63 M. J. L. Sullivan, et al., 'Community-Based Psychosocial Intervention for Musculoskeletal Disorders', *Journal of Occupational Rehabilitation* 15, no. 3 (2005): 377–92.

64 M. O. Martel, et al., 'Catastrophic Thinking and Increased Risk for Prescription Opioid Misuse in Patients with Chronic Pain', *Drug and Alcohol Dependence* 132, no. 1–2 (2013): 335–41.

65 R. R. Edwards, et al., 'Pain-related Catastrophizing as Risk Factor for Suicidal Ideation in Chronic Pain', *Pain* 126, no. 1–3 (2006): 272–9.

66 R. R. Edwards, et al., 'Association of Catastrophizing with Interleukin-6 Responses to Acute Pain', *Pain* 140, no. 1 (2008): 135–44.

67 H. R. Schiphorst, et al., 'Do Analgesics Improve Functioning in Patients with Chronic Low Back Pain?', *European Spine Journal* 23, no. 4 (2014): 800–6.

68 M. M. Vissers, et al., 'Psychological Factors Affecting Outcome of Hip and Knee Arthroplasty', *Seminars in Arthritis and Rheumatism* 41, no. 4 (2012): 576–88.

69 M. O. Martel, et al., 'Association Between Catastrophizing and Craving in Patients with Chronic Pain Prescribed Opioid Therapy', *Pain Medicine* 15, no. 10 (2014): 1757–64.

70 M. J. de Boer, et al., 'Mindfulness, Acceptance and Catastrophizing in Chronic Pain', *PLoS One* 9, no. 1 (2014): e87445.

71 J. W. S. Vlaeyena and S. J. Linton, 'Fear-Avoidance and its Consequences in Chronic Musculoskeletal Pain', *Pain* 85, no. 3 (2000): 317–32.

72 G. Crombez, et al., 'Fear-Avoidance Model of Chronic Pain', *Clinical Journal of Pain* 28, no. 6 (2012): 475–83.

73 G. Crombez, et al., 'Hypervigilance to Pain', *Pain* 116, no. 1–2 (2005): 4–7.

74 S. Morley, 'Psychology of Pain', *British Journal of Anaesthesia* 101, no. 1 (2008): 25–31.

75 S. Volders, et al., 'Avoidance Behaviour in Chronic Pain Research', *Behaviour Research and Therapy* 64 (2015): 31–7.

76 A. L. J. Burke, et al., 'Psychological Functioning of People Living with Chronic Pain', *British Journal of Clinical Psychology* 54, no. 3 (2015): 349–60.

77 N. Buer and S. J. Linton, 'Fear-avoidance Beliefs and Catastrophizing', *Pain* 99, no. 3 (2002): 485–91; M. M. Wertli, et al., 'Fear-avoidance Beliefs: Moderator of Treatment Efficacy in Low Back Pain', *Spine Journal* 14, no. 11 (2014): 2658–78.

78 Crombez, et al., 'Fear-Avoidance Model of Chronic Pain', 476.

79 Edwards, et al., 'Psychosocial Processes in Chronic Pain', T75.

80 N. Afari, et al., 'Psychological Trauma and Functional Somatic Syndromes', *Psychosomatic Medicine* 76, no. 1 (2014): 2–11.

81 K. W. Springer, et al., 'Long-term Health Outcomes of Childhood Abuse', *Journal of General Internal Medicine* 18, no. 10 (2003): 864–70; J. McCauley, et al., 'Clinical Characteristics of Women with a History of Childhood Abuse', *Journal of the American Medical Association* 277, no. 17 (1997): 1362–8; R. T. Goldberg, 'Childhood Abuse, Depression, and Chronic Pain', *Clinical Journal of Pain* 10, no. 4 (1994): 277–81.

82 F. E. Springs and W. N. Friedrich, 'Health Risk Behaviors and Medical Sequelae of Childhood Sexual Abuse', *Mayo Clinical Proceedings* 67, no. 6 (1992): 527–32.

83 M. P. Thompson, et al., 'Association between Childhood Physical, Sexual Victimization and Health Problems in Adulthood', *Journal of Interpersonal Violence* 17, no. 10 (2002): 1115–29.

84 Springer, et al., 'Long-term Health Outcomes of Childhood Abuse'.

85 J. M. Golding, 'Sexual Assault History and Limitations in Physical Functioning', *Research in Nursing and Health* 19, no. 1 (1996): 33–44.

86 N. Sachs-Ericsson, et al., 'Review of Childhood Abuse, Health, and Pain-Related Problems', *Journal of Trauma and Dissociation* 10, no. 2 (2009): 170–88.

87 Springer, et al., 'Long-term Health Outcomes of Childhood Abuse', 864.

88 M. Sharpe and A. Carson, '"Unexplained" Somatic Symptoms', *Annals of Internal Medicine* 134, no. 9 (2001): 926–30.

89 B. A. Arnow, 'Relationships Between Childhood Maltreatment, Adult Health, Psychiatric Outcomes, and Medical Utilization', *Journal of Clinical Psychiatry* 65, no. 12 (2004): 10–15.

90 Sachs-Ericsson, et al., 'Childhood Abuse, Health, and Pain-Related Problems'.

91 K. A. Kendall Tackett, 'Physiological Correlates of Childhood Abuse', *Child Abuse & Neglect* 24, no. 6 (2000): 799–810. See also: I. Timmers, et al., 'The Interaction Between Stress and Chronic Pain', *Neuroscience and Biobehavioral Review* 107 (2019): 641–55.

92 M. Altemus, et al., 'Enhanced Cellular Immune Response in Women with PTSD Related to Childhood Abuse', *American Journal of Psychiatry* 160, no. 9 (2003): 1705–7.

93 H. M. Burke, et al., 'Depression and Cortisol Responses to Psychological Stress', *Psychoneuroendocrinology* 30, no. 9 (2005): 846–56.

94 Arnow, 'Relationships Between Childhood Maltreatment, Adult Health and Psychiatric Outcomes', 13.

95 E. Walker, et al., 'Relationship of Chronic Pelvic Pain to Psychiatric Diagnoses and Childhood Sexual Abuse', *American Journal of Psychiatry* 145, no. 1 (1988): 75–80.

96 J. Jenewein, et al., 'Mutual Influence of Posttraumatic Stress Disorder Symptoms and Chronic Pain', *Journal of Trauma Stress* 22, no. 6 (2009): 540–8.

97 A. Kongsted, et al., 'Acute Stress Response and Recovery after Whiplash Injuries', *European Journal of Pain* 12, no. 4 (2008): 455–63.

98 J. Wuest, et al., 'Chronic Pain in Survivors of Intimate Partner Violence', *Journal of Women's Health* 19, no. 9 (2010): 1665–74; J. Wuest, et al., 'Abuse-Related Injury and PTSD as Mechanisms of Chronic Pain', *Pain Medicine* 10, no. 4 (2009): 739–47.

99 K. G. Raphael and C. Spatz Widom, 'PTSD Moderates Relation between Documented Childhood Victimization and Pain 30 years Later', *Pain* 152, no. 1 (2011): 163–9, 167.

100 J. Tesarz, et al., 'Pain Perception and Processing in Individuals with PTSD', *Pain Reports* 5, no. 5 (2020): e849.

101 K. R. Cromer and N. Sachs-Ericsson, 'Association between Childhood Abuse, PTSD, and Adult Health Problems', *Journal of Trauma Stress* 19, no. 6 (2006): 967–71.

102 L.-A. Mcnutt, et al., 'Cumulative Abuse Experiences, Physical Health and Health Behaviors', *Annals of Epidemiology* 12, no. 2 (2002): 123–30.

103 J. McCauley, et al., 'The "Battering Syndrome": Clinical Characteristics of Domestic Violence', *Annals of Internal Medicine* 123, no. 10 (1995): 737–46; J. McCauley, et al., 'Relation of Low-Severity Violence to Women's Health', *Journal of General Internal Medicine* 13, no. 10 (1998): 687–91.

104 Edwards, et al., 'Psychosocial Processes in Chronic Pain', T77–8.

105 A. V. Apkarian, et al., 'Towards a Theory of Chronic Pain', *Progressive Neurobiology* 87, no. 2 (2009): 81–97; I. Tracey and P. W. Mantyh, 'Cerebral Signature for Pain Perception and its Modulation', *Neuron* 55, no. 3 (2007): 377–91.

106 D. M. Doleys, 'Pain and the Brain', in *Pain: Dynamics and Complexities*, ed. Doleys (Oxford: Oxford University Press, 2014), 43–67.

107 T. Singer, et al., 'Empathy for Pain Involves Affective but not Sensory Components of Pain', *Science* 303, no. 5661 (2004): 1157–62; T. T. Raij, et al., 'Brain Correlates of Subjective Reality of Physically and Psychologically Induced Pain', *Proceedings of the National Academy of Science* 102, no. 6 (2005): 2147–51.

108 A. V. Apkarian, et al., 'Human Brain Mechanisms of Pain Perception and Regulation', *European Journal of Pain* 9, no. 4 (2005): 463–84.

109 P. S. Goldman-Rakic, 'The Prefrontal Landscape', *Philosophical Transactions of the Royal Society of London* 351, no. 1346 (1996): 1445–53.

110 S. Rose, *The Twenty-First Century Brain* (London: Vintage, 2006), 46.

111 M. L. Loggia, et al., 'Lateral Prefrontal Cortex Mediates Hyperalgesic Effects of Negative Cognitions in Chronic Pain', *Journal of Pain* 16, no. 8 (2015): 692–9; W.-Y. Ong, et al., 'Role of Prefrontal Cortex in Pain Processing', *Molecular Neurobiology* 56, no. 2 (2019): 1137–66; D. A. Seminowicz and M. Moayedi, 'Dorsolateral Prefrontal Cortex in Acute and Chronic Pain', *Journal of Pain* 18, no. 9 (2017): 1027–35.

112 A. May, 'Chronic Pain May Change the Structure of the Brain', *Pain* 137, no. 1 (2008): 7–15; F. Cauda, et al., 'Gray Matter Alterations in Chronic Pain', *NeuroImage: Clinical* 4 (2014): 676–86; C. Yuan, et al., 'Gray Matter Abnormalities Associated with Chronic Backpain', *Clinical Journal of Pain* 33, no. 11 (2017): 983–90.

113 A. V. Apkarian, et al., 'Chronic Back Pain associated with Decreased Prefrontal and Thalamic Gray Matter Density', *Journal of Neuroscience* 24, no. 46 (2004): 10410–15; T. Schmidt-Wilcke, et al., 'Affective Components and Intensity of Pain Correlate with Structural Differences in Gray Matter', *Pain* 125, no. 1–2 (2006): 89–97.

114 M. N. Baliki, et al., 'Corticostriatal Functional Connectivity Predicts Transition to Chronic Back Pain', *Nature Neuroscience* 15, no. 8 (2012): 1117–19.

115 R. Rodriguez-Raecke, et al., 'Brain Gray Matter Decrease in Chronic Pain is Consequence and not Cause of Pain', *Journal of Neuroscience* 29, no. 44 (2009): 13746–50.

116 See A. V. Apkarian, et al., 'Pain and the Brain: Specificity and Plasticity of the Brain in Clinical Chronic Pain', *Pain* 152, no. 3 (2011): S49–S64; A. V. Apkarian, 'Pain Perception in Relation to Emotional Learning', *Current Opinion in Neurobiology* 1844 (2008): 464–8.

117 Apkarian, 'Towards a Theory of Chronic Pain', 93.

118 A. Fayaz, et al., 'Prevalence of Chronic Pain in the UK', *BMJ Open* 6, no. 6 (2016): e010364.

119 Mills, et al., 'Chronic Pain: A Review'.

120 I. Gobina, et al., 'Prevalence of Self-Reported Chronic Pain Among Adolescents', *European Journal of Pain* 23, no. 2 (2019): 316e26.

121 H. Breivik, et al., 'Survey of Chronic Pain in Europe', *European Journal of Pain* 10, no. 4 (2006): 287–333.

122 E. J. Bartley and R. B. Fillingim, 'Sex Differences in Pain', *British Journal of Anaesthesia* 111, no. 1 (2013): 52–8.

123 R. M. Craft, et al., 'Sex Differences in Pain and Analgesia', *European Journal of Pain* 8, no. 5 (2004): 397–411; Z. Wiesenfeld-Hallin, 'Sex Differences in Pain Perception', *Gender Medicine* 2, no. 3 (2005): 137–45; N. El-Shormilisy, et al., 'Associations Among Gender: Coping Patterns and Functioning for Individuals with Chronic Pain', *Pain Research Management* 20, no. 1 (2015): 48–55.

124 J. D. Greenspan, et al., 'Studying Sex and Gender Differences in Pain and Analgesia', *Pain* 132, no. 1 (2007): S26–S45.

125 U. John, et al., 'Tobacco Smoking in Relation to Pain', *Preventive Medicine* 43, no. 6 (2006): 477–81.

126 J. W. Ditre, et al., 'Perceived Pain and Tobacco Smoking Interrelations', *Cognitive Behaviour Therapy* 46, no. 4 (2017): 339–51.

127 M. Egli, et al., 'Alcohol Dependence as a Chronic Pain Disorder', *Neuroscience & Biobehavioral Reviews* 36, no. 10 (2012): 2179–92.

128 H. C. Hitt, et al., 'Comorbidity of Obesity and Pain in a General Population', *Journal of Pain* 8, no. 5 (2007): 430–6.

129 G. J. Macfarlane, et al., 'Epidemiology of Common Health Conditions?', *British Journal of Pain* 9, no. 4 (2015): 203–12.

130 F. M. Blyth, 'Chronic Pain-Public Health Problem?', *Pain* 137, no. 3 (2008): 465–6; E. L. Poleshuck and C. R. Green, 'Socioeconomic Disadvantage and Pain', *Pain* 136, no. 3 (2008): 235–8.

131 S. M. Meints, et al., 'Racial and Ethnic Differences in the Experience and Treatment of Noncancer Pain', *Pain Management* 9, no. 3 (2019): 317–34.

132 A. Maly and A. H. Vallerand, 'Neighborhood, Socioeconomic, and Racial Influence on Chronic Pain', *Pain Management Nursing* 19, no. 1 (2018): 14–22.

133 Meints, et al., 'Racial and Ethnic Differences in Noncancer Pain'.

134 W. J. Hall, et al., 'Implicit Racial/Ethnic Bias Among Health Care Professionals', *American Journal of Public Health* 105, no. 12 (2015): e60–e76.

135 T. S. Carey and J. Mills Garrett, 'Relation of Race to Outcomes and Use of Health Care Services for Acute Low Back Pain', *Spine (Phila Pa 1976)* 28, no. 4 (2003): 390–4.

136 D. R. Williams and C. Collins, 'Racial Residential Segregation and Racial Disparities in Health', *Public Health Reports* 116, no. 5 (2001): 404–16.

137 C. M. Campbell and R. R. Edwards, 'Ethnic Differences in Pain and Pain Management', *Pain Management* 2, no. 3 (2012): 219–30; S. A. King, 'Race, Ethnicity and Chronic Pain', *Psychiatric Times* 38, no. 4 (2021): 25.

138 S. H. Meghani, et al., 'Analgesic Treatment Disparities for Pain in the United States', *Pain Medicine* 13, no. 2 (2012): 150–74.

139 C. C. Reyes-Gibby, et al., 'Pain in Aging Non-Hispanic Whites, Non-Hispanic Blacks, and Hispanics', *Journal of Pain* 8, no. 1 (2007): 75–84.

140 R. Wyatt, 'Pain and Ethnicity', *American Medical Association Journal of Ethics* 15, no. 5 (2013): 449–54.

141 William, et al., 'Implicit Racial/Ethnic Bias'; Meints, et al., 'Racial and Ethnic Differences in Noncancer Pain'.

142 S. A. Dugan, et al., 'Chronic Discrimination and Bodily Pain in a Multiethnic Cohort of Midlife Women', *Pain* 158, no. 9 (2017): 1656–65; D. J. Burgess, et al., 'Effect of Perceived Racial Discrimination on Bodily Pain Among Older African American Men', *Pain Medicine* 10, no. 8 (2009): 1341–52.

143 J. L. Walker Taylor, et al., 'Pain, Racial Discrimination, and Depressive Symptoms among African American Women', *Pain Management Nursing* 19, no. 1 (2018): 79–87.

144 O. A. Sotubo, 'Health Inequalities in BAME Communities', *Future Healthcare Journal* 8, no. 1 (2021): 36–9.

145 Breivik, et al., 'Survey of Chronic Pain in Europe'.

146 Banks and Kerns, 'Explaining High Rates of Depression in Chronic Pain'; R. R. Edwards, et al., 'Role of Psychosocial Processes in Chronic Pain'.

147 Breivik, et al., 'Survey of Chronic Pain in Europe'.

148 Banks and Kerns, 'Explaining High Rates of Depression in Chronic Pain'.

149 J. Fuentes, et al., 'Enhanced Therapeutic Alliance Modulates Pain Intensity', *Physical Therapy* 94, no. 4 (2014): 477–89.

150 R. N. Jamison and R. R. Edwards, 'Integrating Pain Management in Clinical Practice', *Journal of Clinical Psychology in Medical Settings* 19, no. 1 (2012): 49–64.

151 S. P. Cohen, et al., 'Chronic Pain', *Lancet* 397, no. 10289 (2021): 2082–97, 2087.

152 See J. Evans, *Philosophy for Life* (London: Rider, 2013).

153 S. Morley, 'CBT for Chronic Pain', *Pain* 152, no. 3 (2011): S99–S106, S100.

154 Jamison and Edwards, 'Integrating Pain Management ', 57.

155 B. E. Thorn and J. W. Burns, 'Treatment Mechanisms in Psychosocial Pain Interventions', *Pain* 152, no. 4 (2011): 705–6.

156 S. Morley, et al., 'Clinical Effectiveness of CBT', *Pain* 137, no. 3 (2008): 670–80; M. R. Naylor, et al., 'Predictive Relationships between Chronic Pain and Negative Emotions', *Comprehensive Psychiatry* 52, no. 6 (2011): 731–6.

157 J. A. Turner, et al., 'Short- and Long-term Efficacy of Brief CBT for Patients with Chronic Temporomandibular Disorder Pain', *Pain* 121, no. 3 (2006): 181–94.

158 J. A. Sturgeon, 'Psychological Therapies for Chronic Pain', *Psychology Research and Behaviour Management* 7 (2014): 115–24, 115.

159 R. J. Gatchel, et al., 'Biopsychosocial Approach to Chronic Pain', *Psychological Bulletin* 133, no. 4 (2007): 581–624, 606.

160 C. Eccleston and G. Crombez, 'Advancing Psychological Therapies for Chronic Pain', *F1000 Research* 6, no. 461 (2017): 1–7.

161 A. C. de Williams, et al., 'Psychological Therapies for the Management of Chronic Pain', *Cochrane Database of Systematic Reviews* 11 (2012): 15.

162 Williams, et al., 'Psychological Therapies for Chronic Pain', 15.

163 Engel, 'Clinical Application of the Biopsychosocial Model', 537.

164 F. Thomas et al., 'How Accessible and Acceptable are Current GP Referral Mechanisms for IAPT for Low-Income Patients', *Journal of Mental Health* 29, no. 6 (2020): 706–11, 708–10.

165 IAPT at 10: Achievements and challenges, https://www.england.nhs.uk/blog/iapt-at-10-achievements-and-challenges/#:~:text=To%20mark%2010%20years%20of,service%20during%20its%20first%20decade (accessed 25 June 2024).

166 H. J. Chatterjee et al., 'Non-Clinical Community Interventions', *Arts & Health* 10, no. 2 (2017): 97–123, 117.

167 'Fair Society, Healthy Lives. The Marmot Review: Strategic Review of Health Inequalities in England Post-2010', https://www.gov.uk/research-for-development-outputs/fair-society-healthy-lives-the-marmot-review-strategic-review-of-health-inequalities-in-england-post-2010 (accessed 25 June 2024).

168 Chatterjee, 'Non-Clinical Community Interventions', 98.

169 Chatterjee, 'Non-Clinical Community Interventions', 117.

170 H. Kerryn, et al., 'Social Prescribing: Where is the Evidence', *British Journal of General Practice* 69, no. 678 (2019): 6–7. See also, Chatterjee, 'Non-Clinical Community Interventions', 114–18.

171 Chatterjee, 'Non-Clinical Community Interventions', 116.

172 R. Poole and P. Huxley, 'Social Prescribing: An Inadequate Response to the Degradation of Social Care in Mental Health', *BJPsych Bulletin* 48, no. 1 (2024): 30–3, 30–2.

173 Thomas, 'How Accessible and Acceptable are Current GP Referral Mechanisms for IAPT for Low-Income Patients', 710.

174 See De-Stress 2, https://destressproject.org.uk/ (accessed 29 June 2024).

175 F. Bu et al., 'Equal, Equitable or Exacerbating Inequalities? Patterns and Predictors of Social Prescribing Referrals in 160,128 UK Patients' (pre-print).

176 V. Sveinsdottir, et al., 'Role of CBT in Management of Chronic Nonspecific Back Pain', *Journal of Pain Research* 5 (2012): 371–80, 376.

Chapter 2

1 D. B. Morris, *The Culture of Pain* (Berkeley: University of California Press, 1991), 29, 34.

2 S. Coakley and K. Kaufman Shelemay, eds., *Pain and its Transformations: The Interface of Biology and Culture* (Cambridge, MA: Harvard University Press, 2007), 1–2.

3 P. De Vlieger, et al., 'Pain Solutions Questionnaire (PaSol)', *Pain* 123, no. 3 (2006): 285–93.

4 L. Bending, *The Representation of Bodily Pain in Late Nineteenth–Century English Culture* (Oxford: Oxford University Press, 2000), 18–20.

5 Bending, *Representation of Bodily Pain*, 28.

6 J. Bourke, *The Story of Pain: From Prayer to Painkillers* (Oxford: Oxford University Press, 2014), 124.

7 J. Moscoso, *Pain: A Cultural History*, trans. S. Thomas and P. House (London: Palgrave Macmillan, 2012), 44.

8 Bourke, *Story of Pain*, 129.

9 Bourke, *Story of Pain*, 89, 90–1.

10 Bourke, *Story of Pain*, 90.

11 K. I. Pargament, et al., 'Religious Coping Efforts as Predictors of Outcomes to Significant Negative Life Events', *American Journal of Community Psychology* 18, no. 6 (1990); R. J. Bulman and C. B. Wortman, 'Attributions of Blame and Coping in the "Real World"', *Journal of Personality and Social Psychology* 35, no. 5 (1977): 351–63.

12 E. A. Rippentrop, et al., 'Relationship between Religion/Spirituality, Physical Health, Mental Health and Pain', *Pain* 116, no. 3 (2005): 311–21; A. M. McCaffrey, et al., 'Prayer for Health Concerns', *Archives of Internal Medicine* 164, no. 8 (2004): 858–62.

13 M. Baetz and R. Bowen, 'Chronic Pain and Fatigue: Associations with Religion and Spirituality', *Pain Research Management* 13, no. 5 (2008): 383–8, 386.

14 A. Büssing, et al., 'Are Spirituality and Religiosity Resources for Patients with Chronic Pain Conditions?', *Pain Medicine* 10, no. 2 (2009): 328–99, 328.

15 E.-M. E. Jegindø, et al., 'Expectations Contribute to Reduced Pain Levels during Prayer', *Journal of Behavioural Medicine* 36, no. 4 (2013): 413–26.

16 J. V. Edwards, et al., 'Self-Management of Chronic Pain: Role of Religious Faith', *Journal of Disability and Religion* 20, no. 44 (2016): 291–306.

17 Bourke, *Story of Pain*, 91.

18 C. Saunders, *Selected Writings: 1958–2004* (Oxford: Oxford University Press, 2006), 166.

19 P.J. Siddall, et al., 'Spirituality: Its Role in Pain Medicine', *Pain Medicine* 16, no. 1 (2015): 51–60, 52.

20 D. Clark, *Cicely Saunders: A Life and Legacy* (Oxford: Oxford University Press, 2018), 29.

21 C. Saunders, 'Evolution of Palliative Care', *Journal of Royal Society of Medicine* 94, no. 9 (2001): 430–2, 430.

22 Clark, *Cicely Saunders*, 34.

23 Clark, *Cicely Saunders*, 44.

24 Clark, *Cicely Saunders*, 50.

25 Saunders, 'Evolution of Palliative Care', 430.

26 Keefe, *Empire of Pain*, 159–62.

27 Saunders, *Selected Writings*, 148.

28 Saunders, 'Evolution of Palliative Care', 431.

29 Clark, *Cicely Saunders*, 109.

30 Saunders, 'Evolution of Palliative Care', 430.

31 C. Saunders, 'Care of Patients Suffering from Terminal Illness', *Nursing Mirror*, 14 February 1964, vii–x.

32 Saunders, *Selected Writings*, 87, 166.

33 C. Saunders, 'Drug Treatment in the Terminal Stages of Cancer', *Current Medicine and Drugs* 1, no. 1 (1960): 16–28, 16.

34 Saunders, *Selected Writings*, 100.

35 D. Clark, 'Total Pain', *Social Science & Medicine* 49, no. 6 (1999): 727–36, 728.

36 Saunders, *Selected Writings*, 87.

37 Saunders, 'Evolution of Palliative Care', 431.

38 Saunders, *Selected Writings*, 243.

39 Saunders, 'Evolution of Palliative Care', 431.

40 Saunders, *Selected Writings*, 97.

41 Saunders, *Selected Writings*, 148.

42 C. Saunders, *Uncertainty and Fear* (London: Queen's Institute of District Nursing, 1962), 8.

43 Clark, 'Total Pain', 733. (See Cicely Saunders, 'And from Sudden Death . . .', *Nursing Times*, 17 August 1962, 1045–46, 1046.)

44 See, for example: M. Cobb, et al., 'Spiritual Needs of Palliative Care Patients', *Journal of Pain and Symptom Management* 43, no. 6 (2012): 1105–19.

45 See Billington, *Is Literature Healthy*, 51–8, 64–71.

46 J.E. Jackson, *Camp Pain: Talking with Chronic Pain Patients* (Philadelphia: University of Pennsylvania Press, 2001), 6.

47 Jackson, *Camp Pain*, 6, 25, 81, 25, 8.

48 Jackson, *Camp Pain*, 8.

49 Jackson, *Camp Pain*, 9, 13.

50 Jackson, *Camp Pain*, 17.

51 Jackson, *Camp Pain*, 17–18, 9.

52 Jackson, *Camp Pain*, 76, 24, 9, 76–7, 86, 78.

53 Jackson, *Camp Pain*, 119–20.

54 Jackson, *Camp Pain*, 120–1.

55 Jackson, *Camp Pain*, 113, 114, 115, 112, 116, 117.

56 W. James, *The Varieties of Religious Experience*, ed. William Proudfoot (New York: Barnes and Noble, 1902/2004), 175–7 (emphasis in original).

57 James, *Varieties of Religious Experience*, 177.

58 James, *Varieties of Religious Experience*, 183, 187.

59 James, *Varieties of Religious Experience*, 207, 209.

Chapter 3

1 Jackson, *Camp Pain*, 8.

2 Jackson, *Camp Pain*, 8.

3 Adapted from S. Freud and J. Breuer, *Studies in Hysteria*, trans. and ed. J. Strachey (1895; London: Hogarth Press, 1957), 135–81.

4 Freud and Breuer, *Studies in Hysteria* (1895), 139.

5 Freud and Breuer, *Studies in Hysteria* (1895), 144.

6 Adapted from Freud and Breuer, *Studies in Hysteria* (1895), 164–6.

7 Freud and Breuer, *Studies in Hysteria* (1895), 168, 157, 166.

8 Freud and Breuer, *Studies in Hysteria* (1895), 8.

9 Freud and Breuer, *Studies in Hysteria* (1895), 117.

10 Freud and Breuer, *Studies in Hysteria* (1895), 161–2.

11 Freud and Breuer, *Studies in Hysteria* (1895), 162–3.

12 Freud and Breuer, *Studies in Hysteria* (1895), 167–8.

13 Freud and Breuer, *Studies in Hysteria* (1895), 168, 152.

14 Freud and Breuer, *Studies in Hysteria* (1895), 169.

15 Freud and Breuer, *Studies in Hysteria* (1895), 173–4.

16 Freud and Breuer, *Studies in Hysteria* (1895), 152.

17 E. Roudinesco, *Why Psychoanalysis?* trans. R. Bowlby (New York: Columbia University Press, 2001), 6–7.

18 R. Bowlby, Introduction to S. Freud and J. Breuer, *Studies in Hysteria*, trans. N. Luckhurst (London: Penguin Books Ltd, 2004), xv.

19 Freud and Breuer, *Studies in Hysteria* (1895), 175.

20 G. E. Engel, '"Psychogenic" Pain and the Pain-Prone Patient', *American Journal of Medicine* 26, no. 6 (1959): 899–918, 916.

21 Engel, '"Psychogenic" Pain', 910, 908, 916.

22 Engel, '"Psychogenic" Pain', 909.

23 Engel, '"Psychogenic" Pain', 911.

24 Engel, '"Psychogenic" Pain', 911.

25 Engel, '"Psychogenic" Pain', 907, 911.

26 Engel, '"Psychogenic" Pain', 916–18.

27 G. J. Taylor, 'Challenge of Chronic Pain: A Psychoanalytic Approach', *Journal of the American Academy of Psychoanalysis and Dynamic Psychiatry* 36, no. 1 (2008): 49–68, 49–50.

28 Taylor, 'Challenge of Chronic Pain', 50.

29 J. Bowlby, *Attachment and Loss*, 3 vols (New York: Basic Books, 1969; London: Hogarth Press, 1973, 1980).

30 L. C. Kolb, 'Attachment Behaviour and Pain Complaints', *Psychosomatics* 23, no. 4 (1982): 413–25, 414.

31 D. J. Anderson and R. H. Hines, 'Attachment and Pain', in *Psychological Vulnerability to Chronic Pain*, ed. R. C. Grzesiak and D. S. Ciccone (New York: Springer, 1994), 137–52, 149.

32 S. F. Mikail, et al., 'An Interpersonally Based Model of Chronic Pain: An Application of Attachment Theory', *Clinical Psychology Review* 14 (1994): 1–16, 11.

33 See especially, P. J. Meredith, 'Attachment Theory and Pain', in *Improving Patient Treatment with Attachment Theory,* ed. J. Hunter and R. Maunder (Cham: Springer, 2016); A. Romeo, et al., 'Attachment Style and Chronic Pain', *Frontiers in Psychology* 8 (2017): 284.

34 T. J. Donnelly and T. Jaaniste, 'Attachment and Chronic Pain in Children and Adolescents', *Children* 3, no. 4 (2016): 21.

35 'Although a number of researchers have made theoretically-derived treatment recommendations for attachment-based interventions for chronic pain such interventions have not been comprehensively outlined, let alone evaluated, within the pediatric chronic pain context.' Donnelly and Jaaniste, 'Attachment and Chronic Pain in Children and Adolescents', 21.

36 S. D. Perlman, 'Psychoanalytic Treatment of Chronic Pain', *Journal of the American Academy of Psychoanalysis* 24, no. 2 (1996): 257–71, 264.

37 S. Ali, et al., 'Conversion Disorder – Mind versus Body', *Innovations in Clinical Neuroscience* 12, no. 5–6 (2015): 27–33.

38 P. Vuilleumier, et al., 'Functional Neuroanatomical Correlates of Hysterical Sensorimotor Loss', *Brain* 124, no. 6 (2001): 1077–90; S. Harvey, et al., 'Conversion Disorder: Towards a Neurobiological Understanding', *Neuropsychiatric Disease and Treatment* 2, no. 1 (2006): 13–20.

39 S. O'Sullivan, *It's All in Your Head: Stories from the Frontline of Psychosomatic Illness* (London: Vintage, 2015), 191. For an understanding of some of the 'shortcomings' and controversy around *Studies in Hysteria*, see Bowlby (2004).

40 O'Sullivan, *It's All in Your Head*, 17.

41 American Psychiatric Association, *Diagnostic and Statistical Manual of Mental Disorders DSM*, 3rd ed. (Washington, DC: American Psychiatric Association, 1980).

42 American Psychiatric Association, *DSM*, rev 3rd ed. (Washington, DC: American Psychiatric Association, 1987).

43 L. Gagliese and J. Katz, 'Medically Unexplained Pain is not Caused by Psychopathology', *Pain Research and Management* 5, no. 4 (2000): 251–7, 252–5.

44 Jackson, *Camp Pain*, 41.

45 O'Sullivan, *It's All in Your Head*, 17.

46 M. Aigner and M. Bach, 'Clinical Utility of DSM-4 Pain Disorder', *Comprehensive Psychiatry* 40, no. 5 (1999): 353–7, 353.

47 American Psychiatric Association, *DSM*, 4th edn. (Washington, DC: American Psychiatric Association, 1994).

48 American Psychiatric Association Division of Research, 'Highlights of Changes from DSM-4 to DSM-5, Somatic Symptom and Related Disorders', *Focus* 11, no. 4 (2013): 525–7, 526.

49 'Highlights of Changes from *DSM*-4 to *DSM*-5', 526.

50 J. Katz, et al., 'Chronic Pain, Psychopathology, and DSM-5', *La Revue Canadienne de Psychiatrie* 60, no. 4 (2015): 160–7, 164, 160, 162.

51 H. Merskey, 'Pain, Psychogenesis, and Psychiatric Diagnosis', *International Review of Psychiatry* 12 (2000): 99–102, 99, 101.

52 R. Kellner, 'Somatization Theories and Research', *Journal of Nervous and Mental Disease* 178, no. 3 (1990): 150–60.

53 A. K. Jana, et al., 'Current Debates over Nosology of Somatoform Disorders', *Industrial Psychiatry Journal* 21, no. 1 (2012): 4–10.

54 Engel, '"Psychogenic Pain"', 917.

55 J. B. Pontalis, *Frontiers In Psychoanalysis: Between the Dream and Psychic Pain*, trans. Catherine Cullen and Philip Cullen (London: The Hogarth Press, 1981), 195.

56 Pontalis, *Frontiers In Psychoanalysis*, 194–6.

57 S. Freud, *Project for a Scientific Psychology*, in *The Standard Edition of the Complete Psychological Works of Sigmund Freud*, vol. 1, ed. J. Strachey, et al. (London: Hogarth Press, 1953), 349–5, 368.

58 S. Freud, *Inhibitions, Symptoms and Anxiety*, trans. Alix Strachey (London: Hogarth Press, 1949), 169.

59 Freud, *Inhibitions, Symptoms and Anxiety*, 166–9.

60 Freud, *Inhibitions, Symptoms and Anxiety*, 170–1.

61 Pontalis, *Frontiers In Psychoanalysis: Between the Dream and Psychic Pain*, 198.

62 S. Freud, 'The Ego and the Id' (1923), *Standard Edition*, vol. 19 (London: Hogarth Press, 1953), 1–66, 25–6.

63 D. W. Winnicott, 'Psychosomatic Illness in its Positive and Negative Aspects', *International Journal of Psychoanalysis* 47 (1966): 510–16, 514–15.

Chapter 4

1 Freud and Breuer, *Studies in Hysteria* (1895), 82–4.

2 E. Scarry, *The Body in Pain: The Making and Unmaking of the World* (Oxford: Oxford University Press, 1985), 5, 54

3 W. Shakespeare, *King Lear, The Complete Works*, eds. Stanley Wells and Gary Taylor (Oxford: Oxford University Press, 1998), 925–35.

4 Engel, '"Psychogenic" Pain', 900.

5 Scarry, *Body in Pain*, 51, 12, 61, 56, 4, 5.

6 Pontalis, *Frontiers In Psychoanalysis*, 199.

7 Scarry, *Body in Pain*, 60, 54.

8 Scarry, *Body in Pain*, 30, 54.

9 Scarry, *Body in Pain*, 55.

10 J. M. G. Le Clezio, 'The Day that Beaumont Became Acquainted with his Pain', in *Fever*, trans. D. Woodward (London: Penguin Books Ltd, 1966/2008), 56–84, 61, 64, 72.

11 Scarry, *Body in Pain*, 54, 36, 45.

12 American Psychological Association, *APA Dictionary of Psychology*, 2nd ed. (Washington, DC: American Psychological Association, 2015).

13 P. E. Sifneos, 'Revalence of "Alexithymic" Characteristics in Psychosomatic Patients', *Psychotherapy and Psychosomatics* 22 (1973): 255–62.

14 G. J. Taylor, 'History of Alexithymia: The Contributions of Psychoanalysis', in *Alexithymia,* ed. O. Luminet, et al. (Cambridge: Cambridge University Press, 2018), 1–16, 1.

15 F. López-Muñoz and F. Pérez-Fernández, 'A History of the Alexithymia Concept and Its Explanatory Models', *Frontiers in Psychiatry* 10 (2020): 1026.

16 Taylor, 'History of Alexithymia', 5.

17 Emotions remained central to Nemiah's and Sifneos's formulations, whereas Marty's and U'Zan's focus was the traditional Freudian concept of psychic energy and excitation in need of discharge by the mental apparatus.

18 López-Muñoz and Pérez-Fernández, 'History of the Alexithymia Concept'.

19 P. D. MacLean, 'Psychosomatic Disease and the "Visceral Brain"', *Psychosomatic Medicine* 11(1949): 338–53, 350. There is evidence from twenty-first century imaging studies that alexithymic people have reduced brain activity in response to emotional imagery: see T. Mantani, et al., 'Reduced Activation of Posterior Cingulate Cortex During Imagery in Subjects with High Degrees of Alexithymia', *Biological Psychiatry* 57, no. 9 (2005): 982–90.

20 J. Ruesch, 'Infantile Personality', *Psychosomatic Medicine* 10 (1948): 134–44, 136.

21 K. Horney, 'Paucity of Inner Experiences' (1952), in *The Unknown Karen Horney,* ed. B. Paris (New Haven: Yale University Press, 2000), 283–94, 284–5.

22 H. Krystal, 'Integration and Self-Healing in Post-Traumatic States: A Ten Year Retrospective', *American Imago* 48, no. 1 (1991): 93–118.

23 H. Krystal, 'Trauma: Considerations of its Intensity and Chronicity', *International Journal of Psychiatry in Clinical Practice* 8, no. 1 (1971): 11–28.

24 Krystal, 'Integration and Self-Healing in Post-Traumatic States', 97, 106–7.

25 R. M. Bagby, et al., 'The Twenty-Item Toronto Alexithymia Scale-I', *Journal of Psychosomatic Research* 38, no. 1 (1994): 23–32.

26 López-Muñoz and Pérez-Fernández, 'History of the Alexithymia Concept'.

27 M. Di Tella and L. Castelli, 'Alexithymia in Chronic Pain Disorders', *Current Rheumatology Reports* 18 (2016): 41; R. V. Aarona, et al., 'Alexithymia in Individuals with Chronic Pain', *Pain* 160, no. 5 (2019): 994–1006.

28 R. Sagar, et al., 'Alexithymia and Depression', *Indian Journal of Psychiatry* 3, no. 2(2021): 127–33.

29 M. A. Lumley, et al., 'Assessment of Alexithymia in Medical Settings', *Journal of Personality Assessment* 89, no. 3 (2007): 230–46.

30 H. Koechlina, et al., 'Role of Emotion Regulation in Chronic Pain', *Journal of Psychosomatic Research* 107 (2018): 38–45.

31 P. Porcelli and G. J. Taylor, 'Alexithymia and Physical Illness: A Psychosomatic Approach', in *Alexithymia*, ed. O. Luminet, et al., (Cambridge: Cambridge University Press, 2018), 105–26.

32 Jackson, *Camp Pain*, 78.

33 M. A. Lumley, et al., 'Relationship of Alexithymia to Pain Severity', *Journal of Psychosomatic Research* 53, no. 3 (2002): 823–30, 823.

34 K. McRae and J. J. Gross, 'Emotion Regulation', *Emotion* 20, no. 1 (2020): 1–9.

35 See note 30 above.

36 A. Bateman and P. Fonagy, eds., *Handbook of Mentalizing in Mental Health Practice*, 2nd ed. (Washington, DC: American Psychiatric Association Publishing, 2019).

37 López-Muñoz and Pérez-Fernández, 'History of the Alexithymia Concept'.

38 Krystal, 'Integration and Self-Healing in Post-Traumatic States', 109.

39 Taylor, 'History of Alexithymia', 5.

40 See Billington, *Is Literature Healthy?*.

41 W. R. Bion, *Second Thoughts* (London: Maresfield Library, 1993), 111.

42 W. R. Bion, *Learning from Experience* (London: Maresfield Library, 1991), 6–7.

43 Bion, *Second Thoughts*, 111, 116.

44 W. R. Bion, *Attention and Interpretation* (London: Maresfield Library, 1970), 106–9.

45 Bion, *Second Thoughts*, 112, 116.

46 Taylor, 'History of Alexithymia', 6.

47 Horney, 'Paucity of Inner Experiencing', 264.

48 H. B. Levine, *Affect, Representation and Language: Between the Silence and the Cry* (London and New York: Routledge, 2022), 47. Levine quotes from A. Green, 'The Primordial Mind and the Work of the Negative', *International Journal of Psychoanalysis* 79 (1998): 649–65, 658. I return to the work of both thinkers in Part II.

49 Bion, *Second Thoughts*, 111.

50 T. H. Ogden, 'On Holding and Containing, Being and Dreaming', *International Journal of Psychoanalysis* 85 (2004): 1349–63, 1357. The metaphor or model is based, as Ogden points out, on Melanie Klein's concept of projective identification.

51 Levine, *Affect, Representation and Language*, 46.

52 See W. R. Bion, *Attention and Interpretation* (London: Maresfield Library, 1993), 6–25.

53 R. Hartke, 'Psychological Turbulence in the Analytic Situation', in *Growth and Turbulence in the Container/Contained,* ed. H. B. Levine and L. J. Brown (New York: Routledge, 2013), 131–48, 132.

54 Ogden, 'On Holding and Containing', 1354.

55 Levine, *Affect, Representation and Language*, 3.

56 Levine, *Affect, Representation and Language*, 48.

57 L. Kahn, *Psychoanalysis, Apathy and the Postmodern Patient* (Abingdon and New York: Routledge, 2018), 63.

58 W. R. Bion, *Learning from Experience* (London: Maresfield Library, 1962), 57.

59 F. Bion, 'The Days of Our Years', in *The Complete Works of W. R Bion*, vol. 15, ed. C. Mawson (London: Karnac, 2014), 91–111, 106.

60 W. R. Bion, *Cogitations* (London: Karnac, 1992), 99.

Chapter 5

1 For a fuller history of the origin and evolution of The Reader, see J. Davis, Introduction, in A. Macmillan, ed., *A Little Aloud* (London: Random House, 2010), 7–20 and J. Davis, 'The Reading Revolution', in *Stop What You're doing and read this!* (London: Vintage Books, 2011), 115–36.

2 J. Billington, 'Reading for Life: Prison Reading Groups in Practice and Theory', *Critical Survey* 23, no. 3 (2012): 67–85; J. Billington, et al., 'A Literature-Based Intervention for Women Prisoners: Preliminary Findings', *International Journal of Prisoner Health* 12, no. 4 (2016): 230–43.

3 C. Dowrick, et al., 'Get into Reading as an Intervention for Common Mental Health Problems', *Journal of Medical Humanities* 38, no. 1 (2012): 15–20.

4 J. Billington, et al., 'A Literature-Based Intervention for Older People Living with Dementia', *Perspectives in Public Health* 133, no. 3 (2013): 165–73; E. Longden, et al., 'Evaluation of Shared Reading Groups for Adults Living with Dementia', *Journal of Public Health* 15, no. 2 (2016): 75–82.

5 S. Hodge, et al., 'Experiences of a Community Reading Project', *Medical Humanities* 33, no. 2 (2007): 100–4; E. Longden, et al., 'Shared Reading: Assessing the Intrinsic Value of a Literature-Based Health Intervention', *Journal of Medical Humanities* 41, no. 2 (2015): 113–20; E. Gray, et al., 'Interpretative Phenomenological (IPA) Analysis of the Experience of Being in a Reader Group', *Arts & Health* 8, no. 3 (2016): 248–61; P. Davis, et al., *What Literature Can Do* (Liverpool: University of Liverpool, 2016).

6 See J. Billington, 'Literature, Reading and Mental Health', in *Palgrave Encyclopedia of the Health Humanities*, ed. P. Crawford, et al. (London: Springer Nature, 2024), which provides a summary overview of this wide field.

7 For a comprehensive compendium of this work, see J. Billington, ed., *Reading and Mental Health* (Cham: Palgrave, 2019), which also offers various articulations of the critical distinction between Shared Reading and Bibliotherapy. For a selection of the work that has grown up contemporaneously in this field or has developed from it, see P. Canning, 'Text World Theory and Real World Readers: From Literature to Life in a Belfast Prison', *Language and Literature* 26, no. 2 (2017): 172–87; E. Troscianko, 'Eating Disorders, Interpretation, and the Case for Creative Bibiliotherapy Research', *Medical Humanities* 44, no. 3 (2018): 201–11; K.I. Skjerdingstad, et al., 'Shared Reading as an Affordance-Nest for Developing Kinesic Engagement with Poetry: A Case Study', *Cogent Arts & Humanities* 6, no. 1 (2019), https://dx.doi.org/10.1080/23311983.2019.1688631; M.M. Kristensen, et al., 'Shared Reading as Mental Health Promotion Among Newly Retired Men', *Nordic Journal of Arts, Culture, and Health* 2 (2020): 107–21; M. Steenberg, et al., 'Facilitating Reading Engagement in Shared Reading', *Poetics Today* 42, no. 2 (2021): 229–51; C.E. Christiansen and A.L. Dalsgard, 'The Day We Were Dogs: Mental Vulnerability, Shared Reading, and Moments of Transformation', *Ethnos* 49, no. 3 (2021): 286–307; T.R. Anderson, 'Regaining Autonomy, Competence, and Relatedness: Experiences of Two Shared Reading Groups for People Diagnosed with Cancer', *Frontiers in Psychology* 13 (2022), https://doi.org/10.3389/fpsyg .2022.1017166; T.M. Tangeraas, 'Moments of Meeting: A Case Study of Shared Reading of Poetry in a Care Home', *Frontiers in Psychology* 13 (2022), https://doi.org/10.3389/fpsyg.2022.965122; T.R. Anderson and F. Hakemulder, 'The Poem Has Stayed with Me: Continued Processing and Impact from Shared Reading Experiences of People Living with Cancer', *Poetics* 102 (2024): 101847.

 8 A reminder that, when quoting, as I do here, directly from primary data gathered for the study, I use italics to distinguish testimony from participants in the study from quotations from published sources. (See Chapter 1, note 10.)

 9 For published findings, see J. Billington, et al., 'Comparative Study of Cognitive Behavioural Therapy and Shared Reading for Chronic Pain', *Journal of Medical Humanities* 43, no. 3 (2016): 155–65.

10 D. Watson, et al., 'Development and Validation of Brief Measures of Positive and Negative Affect: The PANAS Scales', *Journal of Personality and Social Psychology* 54, no. 6 (1988): 1063–70.

11 J. Billington, et al., 'Developing Innovative Qualitative Approaches in Research on Reading and Health', in Billington, *Reading and Mental Health*, 191–240, 196.

12 James, *Varieties of Religious Experience*, 177. (See also Chapter 2, p. 53.)

13 See, for example, A. Jacobs and D. Kuiken eds., *The Handbook of Empirical Studies of Literature* (Berlin: De Gruyter, 2021).

14 T. Eagleton, *Literary Theory: An Introduction* (London: Routledge, 1983), 9.

15 D.S. Miall and D. Kuiken, 'The Form of Reading: Empirical Studies of Literariness', *Poetics* 25, no. 6 (1998): 327–41, 327.

16 D.S. Miall, 'Affect and Narrative', *Poetics* 17, no. 3 (1988): 259–72; E.W. Kneepkens and R.A. Zwaan, 'Emotions and Literary Text Comprehension', *Poetics* 23, no. 1–2 (1994): 125–38; K. Oatley, 'A Taxonomy of the Emotions of Literary Response and a Theory of Identification in Fictional Narrative', *Poetics* 23, no. 1–2 (1994): 53–74; G.C. Cupchik, et al., 'Emotional Effects

of Reading Excerpts from Short Stories by James Joyce', *Poetics* 25, no. 6 (1998): 363–77.

17 Miall and Kuiken, 'Empirical Studies of Literariness', 328.

18 D.S. Miall and D. Kuiken, 'What is Literariness? Three Components of Literary Reading', *Discourse Processes* 28, no. 2 (1999): 121–38, 124.

19 F. Hakemulder, et al. eds., *Narrative Absorption* (Amsterdam: John Benjamins, 2017), 2.

20 H. Bilandzic and R. Buselle, 'Beyond Metaphors and Traditions', in Hakemulder, et al. eds., *Narrative Absorption*, 11–27, 15.

21 P. Davis and J. Billington, 'A Methodology for Literary Reading', in *Edinburgh History of Reading: Modern Readers*, ed. M. Hammond (Edinburgh: Edinburgh University Press, 2020), 283–305; P. Davis and J. Billington, 'Reading', in *The Routledge Companion to Health Humanities*, ed. P. Crawford, et al. (London: Routledge, 2020), 282–6.

22 J. Billington, et al., 'A Literature-Based Intervention for People with Chronic Pain', *International Journal of Arts & Health* 8, no. 1 (2014): 13–31.

23 E. Wharton, 'Mrs Manstey's View', in *Edith Wharton: Collected Stories 1991–1910*, ed. M. Howard (New York: Library of America, 2001), 1–12, 1–4.

24 Wharton, *Collected Stories 1991–1910*, 4–5.

25 D. Kuiken, et al., 'The Experiencing Questionnaire', *Scientific Study of Literature* 2, no. 2 (2012): 243–72, 245.

26 S. Sikora, et al., 'An Uncommon Resonance: the Influence of Loss on Expressive Reading', *Empirical Studies of the Arts* 28, no. 2 (2010): 135–53, 137–9.

27 P. Davis et al., *Assessing the Intrinsic Value of The Reader Organisation's Shared Reading Scheme* (Liverpool: University of Liverpool, 2014), 16–17.

28 K. Oatley, *Such Stuff as Dreams: The Psychology of Fiction* (Oxford: Wiley-Blackwell, 2011), 19.

29 K. Oatley, 'The Mind's Flight Simulator', *The Psychologist*, 10 December 2008.

30 J. Robinson, et al., 'Using Established Qualitative Methods in Research on Reading and Health', in Billington, *Reading and Mental Health*, 155–90.

31 See: Billington, et al., 'Literature-Based Intervention for Women Prisoners' and Canning, 'Text World Theory and Real World Readers'.

32 Billington, 'Prison Reading Groups in Practice and Theory'.

33 Longden, et al., 'Shared Reading: Assessing the Intrinsic Value', 19.

34 Wharton, *Collected Stories 1991–1910*, 3.

35 Wharton, *Collected Stories 1991–1910*, 4.

36 Oatley, *Such Stuff as Dreams*, ix.

37 Gray, 'IPA Analysis of Experience in a Reader Group', 254.

38 D.S. Miall and D. Kuiken, 'Foregrounding, Defamiliarization, and Affect: Response to Literary Stories', *Poetics* 22 no. 5 (1994): 389–407, 390.

39 J. Mukařovský, 'Standard Language and Poetic Language' (1932), quoted in Miall and Kuiken, 'Foregrounding, Defamiliarization, and Affect', 390.

40 V. Shklovsky, *Art as Technique* (1917), quoted in Miall and Kuiken, 'Foregrounding, Defamiliarization, and Affect', 391.

41 Miall and Kuiken, 'Foregrounding, Defamiliarization, and Affect', 392.

42 See, for example, Billington, et al., 'Innovative Qualitative Approaches in Research on Reading and Health'.

43 The quotations from the poem which follow are all from 'Evening', in *The Selected Poetry of Rainer Maria Rilke*, trans. Stephen Mitchell (London: Picador, 1987), 13.

44 Miall and Kuiken, 'Foregrounding, Defamiliarization, and Affect', 394.

45 D.S. Miall and D. Kuiken, 'A Feeling for Fiction: Becoming What We Behold', *Poetics* 30, no. 4 (2002): 221–41, 224–5.

46 Miall and Kuiken, 'Foregrounding, Defamiliarization, and Affect', 394.

47 Miall and Kuiken, 'A Feeling for Fiction', 227.

48 Miall and Kuiken, 'Foregrounding, Defamiliarization, and Affect', 394–5.

49 D. Kuiken, et al, 'Forms of Self-Implication in Literary Reading', *Poetics Today* 25, no. 2 (2004): 171–203, 175.

50 Miall and Kuiken, 'A Feeling for Fiction', 223, 236.

51 Longden, et al., 'Shared Reading: Assessing the Intrinsic Value', 28.

52 Davis et al., *What Literature Can Do*, 19.

53 E.T. Gendlin, *Experiencing and the Creation of Meaning* (Evanston: Northwestern University Press, 1997), 11, 14–15, 1, 71, xi–xii.

54 E.T. Gendlin, 'The New Phenomenology of Carrying Forward', *Continental Philosophy Review* 37, no. 1 (2004): 127–51, 134–5.

55 Kuiken, et al., The Experiencing Questionnaire', 249, 247, 253.

56 D. Kuiken, 'Metaphoricity, Inexpressible Realisations and Expressive Enactment', in Billington, *Reading and Mental Health*, 345–57.

57 Kuiken, et al., 'Forms of Self-Implication in Literary Reading', 179–80, 185.

58 Wharton, *Collected Stories 1991–1910*, 11.

59 E.T. Gendlin, *Focusing* (London: Rider, 2003), 10.

60 H. de Braude, Review of E.T. Gendlin, 'Saying What We Mean: Implicit Precision and the Responsive Order', *Phenomenological Reviews*, 2020.

61 See www.thereader.org.uk and note 1 above.

62 Gendlin, *Experiencing and the Creation of Meaning*, 15.

Chapter 6

1 E. Bowen, 'The Visitor', in *Elizabeth Bowen: Collected Stories* (London: Vintage, 1999): 128–40, 139.

2 J. M. G. Williams, et al., 'Autobiographical Memory Specificity and Emotional Disorder', *Psychological Bulletin* 133, no. 1 (2007): 122–48, 122.

3 C. A. Köhler, et al., 'Autobiographical Memory Disturbances in Depression', *Neural Plasticity* (2015), https://doi.org/10.1155/2015/759139.

4 Williams, et al., 'Autobiographical Memory Specificity', 123,

5 Williams, et al., 'Autobiographical Memory Specificity', 131.

6 Köhler, et al., 'Autobiographical Memory Disturbances in Depression'.

7 Williams, et al., 'Autobiographical Memory Specificity', 133–5, 122.

8 K. Charmaz, *Good Days, Bad Days: The Self in Chronic Illness and Time* (New Brunswick: Rutgers University Press, 1991), 178–82.

9 P. Atkin, *Some of Us Just Fall: On Nature and Not Getting Better* (London: Sceptre, 2023), 185, 172.

10 Charmaz, *Good Days, Bad Days*, 187–90, 178, 243, 199, 206, 231, 235, 233, 238.

11 Bowen, *Collected Stories*, 132.

12 Bowen, *Collected Stories*, 139–40.

13 S. Sikora, et al., 'Expressive Reading: A Phenomenological Study of Readers' Experience of Coleridge's The Rime of the Ancient Mariner', *Psychology of Aesthetics, Creativity, and the Arts* 5, no. 3 (2011): 258–68.

14 Miall and Kuiken, 'A Feeling For Fiction', 238.

15 Kuiken, et al., 'The Experiencing Questionnaire', 251, 252.

16 Charmaz, *Good Days, Bad Days*, 224–6.

17 T. Wolff, 'The Liar', in *Our Story Begins* (London: Bloomsbury, 2008), 36–53, 46–7.

18 P. O. Wilkinson, et al., 'Rumination, Anxiety, Depressive Symptoms and Subsequent Depression in Adolescents at Risk for Psychopathology', *BMC Psychiatry* 13 (2013): 250.

19 M. J. Edwards, et al., 'Thinking about Thinking about Pain: A Qualitative Investigation of Rumination in Chronic Pain', *Pain Management* 1, no. 4 (2011): 311–23.

20 Williams, et al., 'Autobiographical Memory Specificity', 136–7.

21 Charmaz, *Good Days, Bad Days*, 230–6, 210–18.

22 Köhler, et al., 'Autobiographical Memory Disturbances in Depression'.

23 Williams, et al., 'Autobiographical Memory Specificity', 132.

24 Charmaz, *Good Days, Bad Days*, 219.

25 Miall and Kuiken, 'A Feeling for Fiction', 222.

26 Sikora, et al., 'An Uncommon Resonance', 135–53, 136–7.

27 Sikora, et al., 'Uncommon Resonance', 136.

28 Sikora, et al., 'Uncommon Resonance', 150, 142.

29 Kuiken, et al., 'Forms of Self-Implication in Literary Reading', 194.

30 See G. Farrington, 'Right and Wrong', *The Reader* 59 (2015): 79–84, for a description of Mary's response when the study was still underway.

31 E. Taylor, 'Flesh', in *Elizabeth Taylor: Complete Short Stories* (London: Virago, 2012), 521–33, 527, 528.

32 Atkin, *Some of Us Just Fall*, 166.

33 A. Kafer, *Feminist, Queer, Crip* (Bloomington and Indianapolis: University of Indiana Press, 2013), 26, 37–9.

34 E. Samuels, 'Six Ways of Looking at Crip Time', *Disability Studies Quarterly* 37, no. 3 (2017). Accessed 26 June 2024.

35 Kafer, *Feminist, Queer, Crip*, 27, 39–40.

36 Samuels, 'Six Ways of Looking at Crip Time'.

37 The classic structuralist study on the temporalities of narrative is G. Genette, *Narrative Discourse*, trans. J. E. Lewin (Ithaca: Cornell University Press, 1980). For recent work on the ways in which temporality is written into literature about chronic illness, or how a specific narrative genre (science fiction) foregrounds the non-normative relationship to time characteristic of chronic illness and disability, see S. Nance, 'Inhabiting Duration: Contemporary Poetry, Chronic Illness and Environmental Time', *Journal of Literary & Cultural Disability Studies* 17, no. 1 (2023): 59–75; J. Wälivaara, 'Out of Time: Crip Time and Fantastic Resistance', *Science Fiction Research Association* 52, no. 3 (2020): 238–43.

Chapter 7

1 A. Frank, *The Wounded Storyteller* (Chicago: University of Chicago Press, 1997), 1, 5, 25. Frank's thesis has strong affinity with Charmaz's concept of the 'illness chronology' which I discuss in Chapter 8.

2 R. Charon, *Narrative Medicine: Honoring the Stories of Illness* (Oxford: Oxford University Press, 2008), 3.

3 R. Charon, 'How to Listen for the Talk of Pain', in *Encountering Pain*, ed. D. Padfield and J. Zakrzewska (London: UCL, 2021), 40.

4 Charon, *Narrative Medicine*, 10.

5 Charon, 'How to Listen for the Talk of Pain', 42–3.

6 E. Jennings, 'Resemblances', in *The Collected Poems: Elizabeth Jennings*, ed. E. Mason (Manchester: Carcanet Press Ltd, 2012), 68.

7 Jennings, *Collected Poems*, 68.

8 Jennings, *Collected Poems*, 68.

9 J. Steinbeck, *Of Mice and Men* (London: Penguin Books Ltd, 2000), 57.

10 Miall and Kuiken, 'A Feeling for Fiction', *Poetics*, 2002, 229.

11 E. Muir, 'Dream and Thing', in *Collected Poems* (London: Faber & Faber, 1984), 242. (All ensuing quotes from the poem are from this source.)

12 M. Csikszentmihalyi, *Flow: The Psychology of Optimal Experience* (New York: HarperCollins, 1990).

13 D. Perrson, 'Play and Flow in an Activity Group – a Case Study of Creative Occupations with Chronic Pain Patients', *Scandinavian Journal of Occupational Therapy* 3, no. 1 (1996): 33–42.

14 K. Robinson, et al., 'Is Occupational Therapy Adequately Meeting the Needs of People with Chronic Pain?', *American Journal of Occupational Therapy* 65, no. 1 (2011): 106–13.

15 B. A. K. Thissen, et al., 'The Pleasures of Reading Fiction Explained by Flow, Presence, Identification, Suspense, and Cognitive Involvement', *Psychology of Aesthetics, Creativity, and the Arts* 15, no. 4 (2021): 710–24.

16 M. Csikszentmihalyi, *Flow and the Foundations of Positive Psychology* (Dordrecht: Springer, 2014), xv–xvi.

17 Gray, 'IPA Analysis of Experience of a Reader Group', 259.

18 N. Nicholson, 'The Pot Geranium', in *Norman Nicholson: Collected Poems*, ed. Neil Curry (London: Faber & Faber, 2008), 179.

19 Nicholson, *Collected Poems*, 179.

20 Nicholson, *Collected Poems*, 180.

21 Nicholson, *Collected Poems*, 180.

22 See Chapter 1 for the scientific basis for this intuition. For the group leaders further thoughts on change see: Kate McDonnell, 'Reformulating the Self', *The Reader* 65 (2017), 17-27

23 Charon, *Narrative Medicine*, 7.

24 I. Heath, 'Following the Story: Continuity of Care in General Practice', in *Narrative-Based Medicine: Dialogue and Discourse in Clinical Practice*, ed. T. Greenhalgh and B. Hurwitz (London: BMJ Books, 1998), 83–92, 83.

25 Billington et al., 'CBT and Shared Reading for Chronic Pain', 160.

26 J. E. Jackson, 'How to Narrate Chronic Pain? The Politics of Representation', in *Narrative, Pain and Suffering*, ed. D. B. Carr, et al. (Seattle: IASP Press, 2005), 229–41, 231.

27 Charmaz, *Good Days, Bad Days*, 210, 214–15.

28 Charmaz, *Good Days, Bad Days*, 229, 233.

29 R. W. Crump, ed., *Christina Rossetti: The Complete Poems* (London: Penguin Books Ltd, 2001), 50–1, 50.

30 Crump ed., *Rossetti: Complete Poems*, 51.

31 J. Mukařovský, 'Standard Language and Poetic Language' [1932], in *A Prague School Reader on Aesthetics, Literary Structure, and Style*, ed. P. L. Garvin (Washington, DC: Georgetown University Press, 1964), 17–30, 19.

32 Miall and Kuiken, 'What is Literariness?', 127.

33 D. S. Miall, 'Beyond the Schema Given: Affective Comprehension of Literary Narratives', *Cognition and Emotion* 3, no. 1 (1989): 55–78, 74–6.

34 C. Dickens, *A Christmas Carol* (London: Penguin Books Ltd, 1843/2010), 118, 127.

35 Dickens, *A Christmas Carol*, 111.

Chapter 8

1 D. Padfield, et al., *Perceptions of Pain* (Stockport: Dewi Lewis Publishing, 2003), 19–20, 10, 49.

2 D. Padfield, et al., 'Images as Catalysts for Meaning-Making in Medical Pain Encounters: A Multidisciplinary Analysis', *Medical Humanities* 44, no. 2 (2018): 74–81, 76.

3 Padfield, et al., *Perceptions of Pain*, 18.

4 A. Woods, 'The Limits of Narrative: Provocations for the Medical Humanities', *Medical Humanities* 37, no. 2 (2011): 73–8, 73–5.

5 Charmaz, *Good Days, Bad Days*, 229–30.

6 See https://wp.lancs.ac.uk/translatingpain/ and S. Wasson, 'Before Narrative: Episodic Reading and Representations of Chronic Pain', *Medical Humanities* 44, no. 2 (2018): 106–12.

7 Kafer, *Feminist, Queer, Crip*), 27.

8 Atkin, *Some of Us Just Fall*, 166–7, 171–3, 176–7.

9 Charmaz, *Good Days, Bad Days*, 198, 200–1, 207, 213, 224.

10 Padfield, et al., *Perceptions of Pain*, 25.

11 See note 6.

12 Woods, 'The Limits of Narrative', 74.

13 Padfield, et al., *Perceptions of Pain*, 17–18.

14 L. Sheck, 'Mysteriously Standing', in *Captivity* (New York: Alfred A. Knopf, 2007), 41.

15 Miall and Kuiken, 'Foregrounding, Defamiliarization, and Affect', 389–407.

16 Mukařovský, 'Standard Language and Poetic Language', 19.

17 See Chapter 5, p. 86 and note 38.

18 Gendlin, *Experiencing and the Creation of Meaning*, 80, 17, 34, 37.

19 Padfield, et al., *Perceptions of Pain*, 21.

20 Gendlin, *Focusing*, 15–16.

21 Gendlin, *Experiencing and the Creation of Meaning* ,80.

22 Gendlin, *Focusing*, 26–7.

23 Padfield, et al., *Perceptions of Pain*, 21.

24 Sheck, *Captivity*, 41.

25 Sheck, *Captivity*, 41.

26 I quote here from Howard Levine's very helpful definition of Freud's concept in *Affect, Representation and Language*, 41.

27 S. Freud, 'Constructions in Analysis', in *Standard Edition*, vol. xxiii, ed. James Strachey, 258–9, 263, 260.

28 Freud, 'Constructions', 260.

29 Gendlin, *Experiencing and the Creation of Meaning*, 5.

30 Gendlin, *Experiencing and the Creation of Meaning*, 120.

31 Bowen, *Collected Stories*, 128.

32 Bowen, *Collected Stories*, 130.

33 Bowen, *Collected Stories*, 128

34 Bowen, *Collected Stories*, 129.

35 Gendlin, *Experiencing and the Creation of Meaning*, 27.

36 Gendlin, 'New Phenomenology of Carrying Forward', 130.

37 Gendin, *Experiencing and the Creation of Meaning*, 52, 77, 234–5.

38 Freud and Breuer, *Studies in Hysteria* (1895), 6–7.

39 Miall and Kuiken, 'A Feeling for Fiction', 237.

40 Gendlin, *Experiencing and the Creation of Meaning*, 35.

41 S. Freud, 'Remembering, Repeating and Working Through', *Standard Edition* xii (1950): 145–57, 152–3.

42 Steinbeck, *Of Mice and Me*, 91.

43 Woods, 'The Limits of Narrative', 76.

44 Kuiken, et al., 'Forms of Self-Implication in Literary Reading', 180, 185, 182.

45 Woods, 'The Limits of Narrative', 74.

46 Bowen, *Collected Stories*, 129–30.

47 Samuels, 'Six Ways of Looking at Crip Time'..

48 J. Billington, 'Reading for Life: Prison Reading Groups in Theory and Practice', *Critical Survey* 23, no. 3 (2007): 67–85, 77.

49 Gendlin, *Experiencing and the Creation of Meaning*, 34.

50 von Peter, 'The Temporality of "Chronic" Mental Illness', 13–28, 17–19.

51 H. B. Levine, 'The Colourless Canvas: Representation, Therapeutic Action and the Creation of Mind', *International Journal of Psychoanalysis* 93 (2012): 607–29, 609.

52 W. R. Bion, *Transformations: Change from Learning to Growth* (London: William Heinemann Medical Books Ltd, 1963), 150.

53 Levine, *Affect, Representation and Language*, 42.

54 Levine, 'Representation, Therapeutic Action and the Creation of Mind', 609.

55 Levine, *Affect, Representation and Language*, 3, 20, 24, 47, 3, 9.

56 Levine, *Affect, Representation and Language*, 23.

57 W. R. Bion, 'On Arrogance', *International Journal of Psychoanalysis* 39 (1958): 144–5, 146.

58 Levine, *Affect, Representation and Language*, 73, 24–6.

59 See, for example, J. M. Coetzee and A. Kurtz, *The Good Story* (London: Vintage, 2016).

60 Levine, *Affect, Representation and Language*, 26–7.

61 T. H. Ogden, 'Intuiting the Truth of What's Happening: on Bion's "Notes on Memory and Desire"', *The Psychoanalytic Quarterly* 84, no. 2 (2015): 285–306, 294.

62 Bion, *Attention and Interpretation* (1993), 28.

63 Bion, *Transformations*, 147–9.

64 Bion, *Attention and Interpretation*, 27.

65 J. Aguayo and B. Malin eds., *Wilfred Bion: Los Angeles Seminars and Supervision* (London: Karnac, 2013), 11.

66 Gendlin, *Experiencing and the Creation of Meaning*, 5–6.

67 Levine, *Affect, Representation and Language*, 40.

68 T. H. Ogden, 'What's True and Whose Idea Was It?', *International Journal of Psychoanalysis* 84 (2003): 593–606, 593.

69 F. Capello, 'The Buried Harbor of Dreaming, Psychoanalysis and Literature', in *The Wilfred Bion Tradition*, ed. H. B. Levine and G. Civitarese (London: Karnac Books, 2016), 467–88, 472.

70 A. Green, *On Private Madness* (London: Karnac, 1997), 200–201.

71 Bion, *Transformations*, 4–6.

72 H. Racker, *Transference and Countertransference* (London: Karnac Books, 1968), 132.

73 G. J. Zytaruk and J. T. Boulton, eds., *The Letters of D. H. Lawrence*, vol 2 (Cambridge: Cambridge University Press, 1981), 90.

Chapter 9

1 W.R. Bion, 'Experiences in Groups: and Other Papers' (London: Routledge, 1989),77, 53, 98–100.

2 T.H. Ogden, 'Bion's Four Principles of Mental Functioning', *Fort Da* 14, no. 2 (2008): 11–35, 12, 16.

3 Bion, *Experiences in Groups*, 38–40, 48–50, 65, 82, 100, 162.

4 R.D. Hinshelwood, *W. R. Bion as Clinician: Steering Between Concept and Practice* (Abdingdon: Routledge, 2023), 68.

5 Most notably to the church and army. See Bion, *Experiences in Groups*, 107, 156.

6 J. Billington et al., 'A Comparative Study of Cognitive Behavioural Therapy and Shared Reading for Chronic Pain', [Full Report] (Liverpool: University of Liverpool, 2016), 78.

7 Bion, *Experiences in Groups*, 60, 69, 56, 128.

8 E.V. Harsh, 'A Study into Shared Reading Groups, with Specific Relation to Religious Reading', *Frontiers in Psychology* 13 (2022), Accessed 30 June 2024.

9 J. & N. Symington, *The Clinical Thinking of Wilfred Bion* (London: Routledge, 1996), 131–2.

10 Bion, *Learning from Experience*, 42.

11 Bion, *Experiences in Groups*, 52–3.

12 Symington, *The Clinical Thinking of Wilfred Bion*, 127. 'The apparent difference between group psychology and individual psychology is an illusion produced by the fact that the group brings into prominence phenomena that appear alien to an observer unaccustomed to using the group'. Bion, *Experiences in Groups*, 134.

13 Bion, *Experiences in Groups*, 134, 32, 43.

14 Symington, *The Clinical Thinking of Wilfred Bion*, 127.

15 Bion, *Experiences in Groups*, 101.

16 See Chapter 4, p. 69.

17 See Chapter 4, pp. 69–70.

18 Ogden, 'Bion's Four Principles of Mental Functioning', 14.

19 Bion, *Experiences in Groups*, 162.

20 Symington, *The Clinical Thinking of Wilfred Bion*, 131.

21 Bion, *Experiences in Groups*, 89–91.

22 Ogden, 'Bion's Four Principles of Mental Functioning', 20.

23 Bion, *Experiences in Groups*, 52–5.

24 Billington, et al., 'CBT and Shared Reading for Chronic Pain', 163.

25 Bion, *Experiences in Groups*, 61, 52.

26 Hinshelwood, *W. R. Bion as Clinician: Steering Between Concept and Practice*, 60–2.

27 See C. de Bezenac, 'Physiological Measures of Emotional Processes in Reading Experiences', in Billington, *Reading and Mental Health,* 303–20.

28 Billington, et al., 'CBT and Shared Reading for Chronic Pain', 163.

29 Sofia Lampropoulou, et al., 'Linguistic Approaches', in Billington, *Reading and Mental Health,* 241–63, 255–7.

30 Billington, et al., 'CBT and Shared Reading for Chronic Pain', 163.

31 D. Stern, *The Interpersonal World of the Infant* (London: Karnac, 1998), 140, xv–xviii, 156, 57, 141, 146, 142, 157.

32 J. Jaffe, et al., 'Rhythms of Dialogue in Infancy', *Monographs of the Society for Research in Child Development* 66, no. 2 (2001): i–viii, 1–132.

33 B. Beebe, 'My Journey in Infant Research and Psychoanalysis', *Psychoanalytic Psychology* 31, no. 1 (2014): 4–25, 4, 17, 14.

34 B. Beebe, et al., 'The Origins of 12-Month Attachment: A Microanalysis of 4-Month Mother-Infant Interaction', *Attachment and Human Development* 12, no. 1–2 (2010): 3–141, 17.

35 B. Puls, 'Dance Movement Psychotherapy as Influenced by Daniel Stern', *Dance Therapy Collections* 4 (2017): 91–103.

36 J. Davis, 'Groups Reading Aloud for Wellbeing', *The Lancet* 373, no. 9665 (2009): 714–16, 716.

37 Beebe, 'My Journey in Infant Research', 8.

38 E. Larrissy, ed., *W. B. Yeats: The Major Work* (Oxford: Oxford University Press, 2008), 19.

39 Longden, et al., 'Shared Reading: Assessing the Intrinsic Value', 115.

40 Beebe, 'My Journey in Infant Research', 5.

41 C. Trevarthen, 'Making Sense of Infants Making Sense', *Intellectica* 34, no. 1 (2002): 161–88, 161.

42 Davis, et al., 'Assessing the Intrinsic Value of The Reader Organisation's Volunteer Reader Scheme', 35.

43 A. Green, *Key Ideas for a Contemporary Psychoanalysis. Misrecognition and Recognition of the Unconscious*, trans. A. Weller (London: Routledge, 2005), 35.

44 C. Robson, *Heart Beats: Everyday Life and the Memorized Poem* (Princeton: Princeton University Press, 2012), 13.

45 Robson, *Heart Beats*, 5.

46 D. Miall and E. Dissanayake, 'The Poetics of Babytalk', *Human Nature* 14, no. 4 (2003): 337–64, 347–9.

47 E. Dissanayake, 'Prelinguistic and Preliterate Substrates of Poetic Narrative', *Poetics Today* 32, no. 1 (2011): 55–79, 70, 68, 56–7.

48 Miall and Dissanayake, 'Poetics of Babytalk', 344.

49 Dissanayake, 'Prelinguistic and Preliterate Substrates of Poetic Narrative', 70.

50 Miall and Dissanayake, 'Poetics of Babytalk', 354.

51 M. Klein, *Narrative of a Child Analysis* (London: Hogarth, 1961), 318.

52 See Hinshelwood, *Bion as Clinician: Steering Between Concept and Practice*, 30–72.

53 J. Panksepp and C. Trevarthen, 'The Neuroscience of Emotion in Music', in *Communicative Musicality*, ed. Stephen Malloch and Colwyn Trevarthen (Oxford: Oxford University Press, 2009): 105–46, 107–8.

54 Miall and Dissanayake, 'Poetics of Babytalk', 351.

Chapter 10

1 In a study comparing emotional responses to poetry and music cited later in this chapter, the authors conclude that 'whereas music has frequently been acknowledged to be a pancultural phenomenon that has served important social functions from prehistory onwards, it is typically unappreciated that poetry likewise represents an ancient, cross-cultural and emotionally powerful variety within the human communicative and expressive repertoire'. E. Wassiliwizky, et al., 'The Emotional Power of Poetry: Neural Circuitry, Psychophysiology and Compositional Principles', *Social Cognitive and Affective Neuroscience* 12, no. 8 (2017): 1229–40.

2 M. Thompson and L. McCracken, 'Acceptance and Related Processes in Adjustment to Chronic Pain', *Current Pain and Headache Reports* 15. no. 2 (2011): 144–51, 146–7.

3 K. E. Vowles and L. M. McCracken, 'Psychological Flexibility and Traditional Pain Management Coping Strategies', *Behaviour Research and Therapy* 48, no. 2 (2010): 141–6, 141.

4 L. M. McCracken and K. E. Vowles, 'Psychological Flexibility and Traditional Pain Management Strategies', *Journal of Pain* 8, no. 9 (2007): 700–7, 700–1.

5 K. E. Vowles, et al., 'Acceptance and Commitment Therapy for Chronic Pain', *Journal of Contextual Behavioural Science* 3, no. 2 (2014): 74–80, 77.

6 R. W. Bailey, et al., 'Examining Committed Action in Chronic Pain', *Journal of Pain* 17, no. 10 (2016): 1095–104, 1096.

7 K. E. Vowles, et al., 'Acceptance and Values-based Action in Chronic Pain', *Behaviour Research and Therapy* 49, no. 11 (2011): 748–55, 748.

8 Vowles and McCracken, 'Role of Psychological Flexibility', 144.

9 K. E. Vowles, et al., 'The Model Underlying Acceptance and Commitment Therapy for Chronic Pain', *Behaviour Therapy* 45, no. 3 (2014): 390–401, 396.

10 J. Kabat-Zinn, 'Mindfulness-based Interventions in Context: Past, Present, and Future', *Clinical Psychology Science and Practice* 10, no. 2 (2003): 144–56, 145.

11 J. Kabat-Zinn, 'Outpatient Programme for Chronic Pain Patients Based on the Practice of Mindfulness Meditation', *General Hospital Psychiatry* 4, no. 1 (1982): 33–47; J. Kabat-Zinn, et al., 'Clinical Use of Mindfulness Meditation for the Self-Regulation of Chronic Pain', *Journal of Behavioural Medicine* 8, no. 2 (1985): 163–90; J. Kabat-Zinn, et al., 'Four-Year Follow-Up of a Meditation-Based Programme for Chronic Pain', *Clinical Journal of Pain* (1987): 159–73.

12 Kabat-Zinn, 'An Outpatient Programme in Behavioural Medicine for Chronic Pain Patients', 33.

13 See, for example, P. la Cour and M. Peterson, 'Effects of Mindfulness Meditation on Chronic Pain', *Pain Medicine* 16, no. 4 (2015): 641–52; L. Hilton, et al., 'Mindfulness Meditation for Chronic Pain', *Annals of Behavioural Medicine* 51, no. 2 (2017): 199–213.

14 M. H. Majeed, et al., 'Psychotherapeutic Interventions for Chronic Pain', *International Journal of Psychiatry in Medicine* 54, no. 2 (2019): 140–9.

15 J. D. Creswell, et al., 'Neural Correlates of Dispositional Mindfulness during Affect Labeling', *Psychosomatic Medicine* 69, no. 6 (2007): 560–5.

16 F. Zeidan and D. Vago, 'Mindfulness Meditation–Based Pain Relief', *Annals of New York Academy of Science* 1373, no. 1 (2016): 114–27.

17 E. Bilevicius, et al., 'Altered Neural Activity Associated with Mindfulness during Nociception', *Brain Science* 6, no. 2 (2016): 14.

18 C. A. Brown and A. K. P. Jones, 'Meditation Experience Predicts Less Negative Appraisal of Pain', *Pain* 150, no. 3 (2010): 428–38.

19 See Billington et al., 'A Literature-Based Intervention for People with Chronic Pain', 24.

20 L. Yu and L. M. McCracken, 'Model and Processes of Acceptance and Commitment Therapy (ACT) for Chronic Pain', *Current Pain and Headache Reports* 20, no. 2 (2016): 12.

21 La Cour and Peterson, 'Effects of Mindfulness Meditation on Chronic Pain', 650.

22 J. A. Sturgeon, 'Psychological Therapies for the Management of Chronic Pain', *Psychology Research and Behaviour Management* 7 (2014): 115–24, 118.

23 B. van der Kolk, *The Body Keeps the Score: Mind, Brain and Body in the Transformation of Trauma* (London: Penguin Books Ltd, 2015), 47.

24 I am not in a position to judge the criticisms of the book as a work of neuroscience (see, for example, Kristen Martin, '*The Body Keeps the Score* Offers Uncertain Science in the Name of Self-help. It's Not Alone', *The Washington Post,* 2 August 2023, Accessed 28 June 2024). For that reason, I refer to van der Kolk's neuroscientific thesis mostly in summary and as context. I engage extensively with the book's broader thesis here because: firstly, its findings are based on thirty years of clinical practice with people who are chronically ill and these resonate strongly with research in this field cited in Part I and Part II; secondly, the book's argument as to treatment offers (implicitly) a strong challenge to the notion of therapeutic reading, which challenge rests on ideas of embodiment emerging from Van der Kolk's extensive clinical experience as much as on as the neuroscience the book espouses.

25 Van der Kolk, *The Body Keeps the Score*, 2–3.

26 J. LeDoux, *The Emotional Brain* (London: Phoenix, 2004), 164–6.

27 Van der Kolk, *The Body Keeps the Score*, 204, 96, 21, 53.

28 Van der Kolk, *The Body Keeps the Score*, 21, 190, 43.

29 Van der Kolk, *The Body Keeps the Score*, 43–7, 21.

30 Van der Kolk, *The Body Keeps the Score*, 266–73.

31 B. K. Hölzel, et al., 'Mindfulness Practice Leads to Increases in Regional Brain Gray Matter Density', *Psychiatry Research* 191, no. 1 (2011): 36–43.

32 C. Villemure, et al., 'Insular Cortex Mediates Increased Pain Tolerance in Yoga Practitioners', *Cerebral Cortex* 24, no. 10 (2014): 2732–40.

33 Van der Kolk, *The Body Keeps the Score*, 56, 221, 47.

34 Van der Kolk, *The Body Keeps the Score*, 257–62, 70.

35 Davis and Billington, 'A Methodology for Literary Reading', 283–305, 287.

36 J. Billington, et al., 'Qualitative Methods II: Developing Innovative Qualitative Approaches in Research on Reading and Health', in Billington, ed. *Reading and Mental Health*, 194, 208.

37 D. Fearnley and G. Farrington, 'Reading and Psychiatric Practices', in Billington, *Reading and Mental Health,* 323–19, 327.

38 Longden et al., 'Shared Reading: Assessing the Intrinsic Value', 115.

39 J. Billington and M. Steenberg, 'Literary Reading and Mental Wellbeing', in Jacobs and Kuiken, *Handbook of Empirical Studies of Literature*, 402.

40 Billington, et al. 'Developing Innovative Qualitative Approaches in Research on Reading and Health', 208.

41 Van der Kolk, *The Body Keeps the Score*, 349.

42 Quoted in Billington, *Is Literature Healthy,* 98.

43 Surveying the neuroscientific and clinical evidence from Paul MacLean to Joseph LeDoux, Laura Otis remarks: 'human emotions emerged from cross-talk among many brain regions, those that assessed bodily feedback and those that evaluated meaning in context', 'Affective Neuroscience', in *The Routledge Companion to Literature and Emotion,* ed. P. Hogan, et al. (London: Routledge, 2022), 15–25, 17.

44 Van der Kolk, *The Body Keeps the Score*, 205.

45 A .Phillips, *Side Effects* (London: Hamish Hamilton, 2006), 2, 17.

46 Van der Kolk, *The Body Keeps the Score*, 253.

47 Fearnley and Farrington, 'Reading and Psychiatric Practices', 327.

48 G. Farrington, et al., 'Reading in Clinical Contexts', in Billington, *Reading and Mental Health,* 135–51, 150.

49 V. Gallese and H. Wojciehowski, 'How Stories Make Us Feel: Toward An Embodied Narratology', *California Italian Studies* 2, no. 1 (2011), https://doi.org/10.5070/C321008974.

50 A. Damasio, *Descartes' Error: Emotion, Reason, and the Human Brain* (New York: Penguin Books, 1995), 154.

51 H. Wojciehowski and V. Gallese, 'Embodied Simulation and Emotional Engagement With Fictional Characters', in Hogan, et al., *Routledge Companion to Literature and Emotion,* 61–73, 63.

52 For a full survey of emotion research in cognitive literary studies, see Mario Carraciolo, 'Literary Emotions From Appraisal to Embodiment', in Hogan, et al., *Routledge Companion to Literature and Emotion,* 50–60.

53 Gallese and Wojciehowski, 'How Stories Make Us Feel'.

54 Wassiliwizky, et al., 'The Emotional Power of Poetry', 1237, 1231, 1235.

55 Davis, et al., 'Cultural Value: Assessing the Intrinsic Value of The Reader Organization's Shared Reading Scheme', 10.

56 Wassiliwizky, et al., 'Emotional Power of Poetry', 1238.

57 A. M. Jacobs, 'Neurocognitive Poetics: Methods and Models for Investigating the Neuronal and Cognitive-Affective Bases of Literature Reception', *Frontiers in Human Neuroscience* 16, no. 9 (2015), https://doi.org/10.3389/fnhum.2015.00186. See also A. M. Jacobs, 'Towards a Neurocognitive Poetics Model of Literary Reading', in *Towards a Cognitive Neuroscience of Natural Language Use,* ed. R. Willems (Cambridge: Cambridge University Press, 2015), 135–59.

58 W. Shakespeare, *The Complete Works,* ed. Stanley Wells and Gary Taylor (Oxford: Oxford University Press, 1998), 931.

59 P. Davis, et al., 'Reading: Brain, Mind and Body', in Billington, *Reading and Mental Health,* 295.

60 See P. Davis, et al., 'Event-Related Potential Characterisation of the Shakespearean Functional Shift', *NeuroImage* 40, no. 2 (2008): 923–31; P. Davis, et al., 'How Shakespeare Tempests the Brain', *Cortex* 49, no. 4 (2012): 21–64.

61 A. Feizerfan and G. Sheh, 'Transition from Acute to Chronic Pain', *Continuing Education in Anaesthesia Critical Care & Pain* 15, no. 2 (2015): 98–102, 100–1.

62 N. O'Sullivan, et al., 'The Neural Basis of Literary Awareness and the Benefits to Cognition', *Cortex* 73 (2015): 144–57, 152–4.

63 Lisa Barrett Feldman, *How Emotions Are Made* (London: Macmillan, 2017): 32, xi–xiii, 15–16, 59, 27–31, 82-3, 156, 180–2.

64 Barrett, *How Emotions Are Made*, 28.

65 Keith Oatley, 'Fiction as Cognitive and Emotional Simulation', *Review of General Psychology* 3, no. 2 (1999): 101–17, 108.

66 Barrett, *How Emotions Are Made*, 181.

67 Barrett, *How Emotions Are Made*, 31–3.

68 Barrett, *How Emotions Are Made*, 121, 241.

69 Peter, 'The Temporality of "Chronic" Mental Illness', 19.

70 Levine, *Affect, Representation and Language*, 48, 3.

71 Levine, *Affect, Representation and Language*, 3.

72 Longden, et al., 'Intrinsic Value of a Literature-Based Intervention', 113.

73 Van der Kolk, *The Body Keeps the Score*, 78, 166, 122, 129, 141–2.

74 Barrett, *How Emotions Are Made*, 153–5.

75 Jaak Panksepp, *Affective Neuroscience* (Oxford: Oxford University Press, 1998), 254–5.

76 Barrett, *How Emotions Are Made*, 152.

Afterword

1 Chatterjee, 'Non-Clinical Community Interventions', 117–18.

2 See De-Stress 2, https://destressproject.org.uk/(accessed 29 June 2024).

3 A. Woods and J. Rákóczi, 'Literature in the Critical Medical Humanities', in *Literature and Medicine*, ed. A.M. Elsner and M. Pietrzak-Franger (Cambridge: Cambridge University Press, 2024), 357–74, 360–1, 366, 374.

4 V. J. Camden, [Chronology and] Introduction to *The Cambridge Companion to Literature and Psychoanalysis* (Cambridge: Cambridge University Press, 2022), [xv–xxi], 1–17, [xv], 3–4.

5 Woods and Rákóczi, 'Literature in the Critical Medical Humanities', 374.

6 Jackson, *Camp Pain*, 90.

7 Gendlin, *Experiencing and the Creation of Meaning*, 15–16.

8 P. Fonagy et al., 'Pragmatic Randomized Controlled Trial of Long-Term Psychoanalytic Psychotherapy for Treatment-Resistant Depression: The Tavistock Adult Depression Study (TADS)', *World Psychiatry* 14, no. 3 (2015): 312–21.

9 Peter, 'The Temporality of "Chronic" Mental Illness', 17, 20, 15.

10 Jackson, 'How to Narrate Chronic Pain', 239.

11 K. Burke, *The Philosophy of Literary Form* (Berkeley: University of California Press, 1973), 1–2.

Select Bibliography

Beebe, B. 'My Journey in Infant Research and Psychoanalysis: Microanalysis'. *Psychoanalytic Psychology* 31, no. 1 (2014): 4–25.

Beebe, B., et al. 'The Origins of 12-Month Attachment: A Microanalysis of 4-Month Mother-Infant Interaction'. *Attachment and Human Development* 12, no. 1–2 (2010): 3–141.

Bending, L. *The Representation of Bodily Pain in Late Nineteenth–Century English Culture.* Oxford: Oxford University Press, 2000.

Billington, J., ed. *Reading and Mental Health.* Cham: Palgrave, 2019.

Billington, J., et al. 'A Comparative Study of Cognitive Behavioural Therapy and Shared Reading for Chronic Pain'. *Journal of Medical Humanities* 43, no. 3 (2016): 155–65.

Bion, W. R. *Learning from Experience.* London: Maresfield Library, 1962.

Bion, W. R. *Transformations: Change from Learning to Growth.* London: William Heinemann Medical Books Ltd, 1963.

Bion, W. R. *Experiences in Groups: And Other Papers.* London: Routledge, 1989, 77, 53, 98–100.

Bion, W. R. *Attention and Interpretation.* London: Maresfield Library, 1993.

Bion, W. R. *Second Thoughts.* London: Maresfield Library, 1993.

Bourke, J. *The Story of Pain: From Prayer to Painkiller.* Oxford: Oxford University Press, 2014.

Charmaz, K. *Good Days, Bad Days: The Self in Chronic Illness and Time.* New Brunswick: Rutgers University Press, 1991.

Charon, R. *Narrative Medicine: Honoring the Stories of Illness.* Oxford: Oxford University Press, 2008.

Clark, D. *Cicely Saunders: A Life and Legacy.* Oxford: Oxford University Press, 2018.

Coakley, S. and K. Kaufman Shelemay, eds. *Pain and its Transformations: The Interface of Biology and Culture.* Cambridge, MA: Harvard University Press, 2007.

Csikszentmihalyi, M. *Flow: The Psychology of Optimal Experience.* New York: HarperCollins, 1990.

Dissanayake, E. 'Prelinguistic and Preliterate Substrates of Poetic Narrative'. *Poetics Today* 32, no. 1 (2011): 55–79.

Engel, G. E. '"Psychogenic" Pain and the Pain-Prone Patient'. *American Journal of Medicine* 26, no. 6 (1959): 899–918.

Frank, A. *The Wounded Storyteller.* Chicago: University of Chicago Press, 1997.

Freud, S. and J. Breuer. *Studies in Hysteria.* Translated and edited by J. Strachey. 1895; London: Hogarth Press, 1957.

Gendlin, E. T. *Experiencing and the Creation of Meaning: A Philosophical and Psychological Approach to the Subjective*. Evanston: Northwestern University Press, 1997.

Jackson, J. E. *Camp Pain:Talking with Chronic Pain Patients*. Philadelphia: University of Pennsylvania Press, 2001.

James, W. *Varieties of Religious Experience*. Edited by M. E. Marty. Harmondsworth: Penguin Books Ltd, 1985.

Keefe, P. R. *Empire of Pain*. London: Picador, 2021.

Kleinman, A. *The Illness Narratives: Suffering, Healing and the Human Condition*. New York: Basic Books, 1988.

Krystal, H. 'Integration and Self-Healing in Post-Traumatic States: A Ten Year Retrospective'. *American Imago* 48, no. 1(1991): 93–118.

Kuiken, D., et al. 'Forms of Self-Implication in Literary Reading'. *Poetics Today* 25, no. 2 (2004): 171–203.

Levine, H. B. *Affect, Representation and Language: Between the Silence and the Cry*. London and New York: Routledge, 2022.

Miall, D. S. 'Beyond the Schema Given: Affective Comprehension of Literary Narratives'. *Cognition and Emotion* 3, no. 1 (1989): 55–78.

Miall, D. S. and E. Dissanayake. 'The Poetics of Babytalk'. *Human Nature* 14, no. 4 (2003): 337–64.

Miall, D. S. and D. Kuiken. 'Foregrounding, Defamiliarization, and Affect: Response to Literary Stories'. *Poetics* 22, no. 5 (1994): 389–407.

Miall, D. S. and D. Kuiken. 'What is Literariness? Three Components of Literary Reading'. *Discourse Processes* 28, no. 2 (1999): 121–38.

Miall, D. S. and D. Kuiken. 'A Feeling for Fiction: Becoming What We Behold'. *Poetics* 30, no. 4 (2002): 221–41.

Morris, D. B. *The Culture of Pain*. Berkeley: University of California Press, 1991.

Oatley, K. *Such Stuff as Dreams: The Psychology of Fiction*. Oxford: Wiley-Blackwell, 2011.

Ogden, T. H. 'On Holding and Containing, Being and Dreaming'. *International Journal of Psychoanalysis* 85 (2004): 1349–63.

Padfield, D., et al. *Perceptions of Pain*. Stockport: Dewi Lewis Publishing, 2003.

Paris, B., ed. *The Unknown Karen Horney*. New Haven: Yale University Press, 2000.

Pontalis, J. B. *Frontiers In Psychoanalysis: Between the Dream and Psychic Pain*. Translated by Catherine Cullen and Philip Cullen. London: The Hogarth Press, 1981.

Robson, C. *Heart Beats: Everyday Life and the Memorized Poem*. Princeton: Princeton University Press, 2012.

Roudinesco, E. *Why Psychoanalysis?* Translated by R. Bowlby. New York: Columbia University Press, 2001.

Saunders, C. *Selected Writings: 1958-2004*. Oxford: Oxford University Press, 2006.

Scarry, E. *The Body in Pain: The Making and Unmaking of the World*. New York and Oxford: Oxford University Press, 1985.

Sikora, S., et al. 'An Uncommon Resonance: The Influence of Loss on Expressive Reading'. *Empirical Studies of the Arts* 28, no. 2 (2010): 135–53.

Sikora, S., et al. 'Expressive Reading: A Phenomenological Study of Readers' Experience of Coleridge's The Rime of the Ancient Mariner'. *Psychology of Aesthetics, Creativity, and the Arts* 5, no. 3 (2011): 258–68.

Stern, D. *The Interpersonal World of the Infant: A View from Psychoanalysis and Developmental Psychology.* London: Karnac, 1998.

Van der Kolk, B. *The Body Keeps the Score: Mind, Brain and Body in the Transformation of Trauma.* London: Penguin Books Ltd, 2015.

Wasson, S. 'Before Narrative: Episodic Reading and Representations of Chronic Pain'. *Medical Humanities* 44, no. 2 (2018): 106–12.

Williams, J. M. G., et al. 'Autobiographical Memory Specificity and Emotional Disorder'. *Psychological Bulletin* 133, no. 1 (2007): 122–48.

Woods, A. 'The Limits of Narrative: Provocations for the Medical Humanities'. *Medical Humanities* 37, no. 2 (2011): 73–8.

Index